LANGUAGES AND LINGUISTICS

SPEECH, LANGUAGE AND VOICE PATHOLOGY

METHODS, CHALLENGES AND OUTCOMES

LANGUAGES AND LINGUISTICS

Additional books in this series can be found on Nova's website under the Series tab.

Additional e-books in this series can be found on Nova's website under the e-book tab.

LANGUAGES AND LINGUISTICS

SPEECH, LANGUAGE AND VOICE PATHOLOGY

METHODS, CHALLENGES AND OUTCOMES

PABLO ANTONIO YSUNZA
EDITOR

nova publishers
New York

For permission to use material from this book please contact us:
Telephone 631-231-7269; Fax 631-231-8175
Web Site: http://www.novapublishers.com

Additional color graphics may be available in the e-book version of this book.

Library of Congress Cataloging-in-Publication Data

ISBN: 978-1-63321-958-8

Published by Nova Science Publishers, Inc. † New York

CONTENTS

PREFACE

Speech & Language Pathology is a general term which includes the study of several functions and disorders. Normal linguistic development, developmental language disorders, acquired language disorders, normal speech development, speech impairment, speech and voice disorders associated with craniofacial anomalies, normal swallowing mechanism, swallowing disorders, physiology of voice production and voice disorders among other topics are all addressed in Speech & Language Pathology programs. Therefore, it seems that the term "Speech & Language Pathology" comes short for describing the vast field of knowledge encompassed in this area. Speech, Language and Voice Pathology seems more appropriate. However, even this term does not mention swallowing. Since in semantics "*use becomes rule*", it is probably better to keep using the term "Speech & Language Pathology" but it should be considered that there are functions and pathologies that go beyond this denomination.

The aim of this book is to provide the readers with interesting and useful data concerning several topics in Speech & Language Pathology. Thus, the selected title was Speech, Language and Voice Pathology: Methods, Challenges and Outcomes. It should be emphasized again that swallowing is an important element in Speech & Language Pathology. Moreover, as it will be described later, one of the chapters is actually devoted to the role of the Speech & Language Pathology professional in the management of swallowing disorders in the critical patient.

Two of the chapters of this book are dedicated to speech disorders in craniofacial anomalies, specifically cleft palate. One of the chapters provides an updated review of the diagnosis and classification of compensatory articulation errors and how some strategies of speech intervention can be used for remediating these abnormal articulation patterns. The second chapter addresses a protocol for the management of a residual velopharyngeal insufficiency following initial repair of a palatal cleft in young adults.

Speech & Language Pathology interventions for treating swallowing disorders in patients in critical care are addressed in another chapter. The importance of an early approach in these cases is thoroughly described. As mentioned herein, treating swallowing disorders is definitely within the scope of practice of the Speech & Language Pathology professional.

One of the chapters describes the rationale of using a toolkit for early language intervention in children. In this chapter, how to ensemble a toolkit to be used during speech pathology treatment sessions is described. Although this information may be especially valuable for professionals who are starting to practice, it will also be interesting and useful for experienced Speech & Language Pathologists.

A new speech sound disorders protocol guide for Speech & Language Pathology professionals is presented in another chapter. A thorough review of speech sound disorders and the importance of approaching the diagnosis and management of these disorders through a previously planned and standardized protocol is described and discussed.

The chapter concerning the report of clinical outcomes in Speech & Language Pathology reports the results after twenty years of developing, collecting and analyzing clinical outcomes. Adult and childhood outcomes acquired from the Beaumont Outcome Software System© (BOSS) and the National Outcomes Measurement System (NOMS) of the American Speech-Language Hearing Association are reported in detail. Positive and negative lessons learned from collecting and analyzing clinical outcomes are discussed.

Voice disorders caused by vocal abuse and misuse, their diagnosis and management are addressed in another chapter. The findings of several recent systematic reviews are described and analyzed. The readers will find that this information will be useful for their clinical practice.

Finally, a Meta – analysis of the Impact of Protracted Phonological Disorders on Literacy Outcomes in Children is presented in one of the chapters. The chapter describes how in both initial and later phases of childhood literacy, early spoken phonological intervention seems to be relevant for mitigating differences between children with and without phonological disorders.

In sum, Speech, Language and Voice Pathology: Methods, Challenges and Outcomes presents current and updated points of view about speech related aspects of craniofacial anomalies; phonological disorders; materials for providing Speech & Language Pathology treatments; swallowing disorders in critical care; voice disorders caused by vocal abuse and misuse; a protocol for assessing and treating speech sound disorders; and outcome analysis of Speech & Language Pathology treatments.

In: Speech, Language and Voice Pathology ISBN: 978-1-63321-958-8
Editor: Pablo Antonio Ysunza

Chapter 1

EFFECTIVENESS OF VOICE THERAPY IN VOCAL FOLD NODULES

Victor Valadez*[*] *and Rosa Isela Magallanes
Instituto Nacional de Rehabilitación, Mexico City, Mexico

ABSTRACT

Vocal fold nodules are a functional voice disorder associated with voice misuse and abuse. They are benign masses, typically located on the membranous aspect of the vocal fold. Voice therapy is a process that aims to bring voice to a level of fitness that can supply occupational, emotional and social needs, knowing that not all patients will achieve a normal voice. Voice training usually consists of a combination of "direct" and "indirect" treatment techniques. Direct techniques focus on the underlying physiological changes needed to improve an individual´s technique in using the vocal system. These techniques are aimed to modify and/or improve vocal fold closure (adduction), respiratory patterns, resonance, pitch and articulatory tension. In contrast, indirect procedures concentrate on contributory and maintenance aspects of the voice disorder and may involve relaxation strategies, counselling and explanation of the normal anatomy and physiology of the vocal tract, explanation of the casual factors of voice disorders and voice care and conservation.

---

[*] vvaladez@inr.gob.mx or vicman71_@hotmail.com.

Keywords: Vocal Folds, Vocal cords, Vocal nodules, Voice, Rehabilitation, Therapy

INTRODUCTION

Vocal fold nodules are a functional voice disorder associated with voice misuse and abuse. They are benign masses, typically located on the membranous aspect of the vocal folds. Common symptoms include hoarseness, breathiness, vocal fatigue, straining, rough voice and vocal range decline. [1, 2]

Vocal nodules are a frequently occurring type of voice disorder. Their incidence appears to be related with occupation. [3]

Voice therapy can be conceptualized as a process aiming to bring voice to a level of fitness which can be considered achievable by the patient. This level of improvement should be enough to supply the patient's emotional, social and occupational needs. It should be pointed out that not all patients can achieve an entirely normal voice. [4]

Voice therapy usually starts from awareness of the voice disorder. However, when children exhibit voice disorders, it is quite difficult for them to be aware of their voice abnormal voice quality or their vocal symptoms. [5, 6] Thus, in these cases working with the family becomes essential.

Several authors have reported that vocal treatment of dysphonia, whether organic or functional, can address several aspects which may be applicable to most cases. These include relaxation exercises, breathing exercises and voice projection and impost. [4]

Holmberg, et al [3] reports that clinicians use a variety of therapy approaches to treat vocal nodules. A main goal of the treatment techniques is to reduce muscle tension and hyperfunction and optimize vocal behavior to reduce the trauma to the vocal folds, so that aerodynamic forces and acoustic properties approach normal values. The realm of the therapy can be divided into four basic approaches: 1. vocal hygiene; 2. direct facilitation; 3. Relaxation; and 4. respiration. In addition, it is generally agreed that some time should be devoted to "carryover" newly learned vocal behaviors to "real life" situations outside the therapy setting. Perceptual judgments have long been the major clinical tool for voice evaluation. The clients seek treatment in part because their voice does not sound normal. Speech clinicians use both formal and informal perceptual judgments in each session with the client, and perceptual judgments always serve as a complement to visual inspection of the larynx and vocal folds. In addition, perceptual parameters are used as standards against which objective measures of voice are evaluated. It has been a problem that large intra - listener and inter - listener variations have been found in perceptual evaluations, which therefore have been criticized as being too subjective to have real clinical value. In contrast, good agreements among listeners have been shown in other studies. Much of the recent research reports have focused on objective measurements of vocal function. Unfortunately, the techniques for obtaining such signals are not always easily accessible in clinical centers. Moreover, analyses and interpretations of the results are not straightforward. Identifying voice quality parameters that reflect underlying vocal function should have strong clinical value.

An important goal is to develop reliable methods for perceptual evaluations of voice quality, and to establish reliable relationships between perceptual judgments and objective measures of underlying physiological conditions.

Endoscopic findings have demonstrated vocal hyperfunction in patients with vocal nodules undergoing behaviorally based voice therapy. [3] Based on these findings, it has been possible to define relationships between therapy approaches and desired modifications in vocal function which can be assessed and detected by selected voice quality parameters, hence contributing to the development of perceptual criteria for evaluating treatment outcomes in cases of vocal nodules. At the onset of voice intervention, no differences have been found between evaluations of patients' recordings that have been repeatedly examined for reliability. However, after the intervention period, it has been demonstrated that nodules decreased in size either bilaterally or unilaterally. Also, it has been reported that the surrounding edema that can be found at the onset of voice intervention either unilaterally or bilaterally is significantly decreased after intervention.

In a previous report [3] mean values were always high ($\alpha > 0.80$) for the parameters: press, breathiness, lack of sonority, scrape, and dysphonia, while mean α for other parameters varied across assessments. Strong ($r > 0.70$) positive correlations were found in several assessments between press and gratings; roughness and scrape; and between breathiness and aphonic instances, including lack of sonority and instability. Vocal fry was not strongly correlated with any of the other parameters, but a few cases of significant negative correlations were found between vocal fry and breathiness and aphonic instances. Overall dysphonia before and after therapy was strongly correlated with press, breathiness, and scrape. No cases of significant correlations were found between press and breathiness. Endoscopic ratings of vocal status showed that none of the vocal nodules had completely disappeared after completion of the therapy. This finding is in agreement with histologic studies that suggest that more permanent types of tissue damage may be associated with the formation of nodules, e.g., fibroblastic response involving increased fibronectin decomposition. Thus, the positive impact of therapy is not necessarily associated with a complete amelioration of the nodular lesions. However, the fact that the nodules had decreased in size after therapy for most patients, as well as findings of reduce edema, strongly suggest that voice therapy has a trauma-reducing effect for the majority of patients. Hyperfunctional vocal behavior appears to have decreased. Thus, there seemed to be a good potential that the compensatory “vicious circle” of further increased muscle tension and increased subglottal pressure leading to escalating trauma could be stopped by voice therapy. The combined results from endoscopic and perceptual evaluations suggest that alterations in vocal status and voice function were reflected in parameters of voice quality. These results of decreased nodules and improved voice quality suggest that the voice therapy had a positive effect for a majority of the patients with vocal nodules.

A Cochrane’s systematic review [7] reports that that voice training usually consists of a combination of “direct” and “indirect” treatment techniques. Direct techniques focus on the underlying physiological changes needed to improve an individual´s technique for using the vocal system. These techniques are aimed to modify several functions or behaviors including: vocal fold closure (adduction); respiratory patterns; resonance; pitch; and articulatory tension. In practice this means to guide intensive training concerning modifications of correct posture, breathing techniques and the production of various sounds like humming, singing musical scales or yawing. Indirect techniques, on the other hand, concentrate on contributory and maintenance aspects of the voice disorder and may involve relaxation strategies; counseling; explanation of the normal anatomy and physiology of the vocal tract; explanation of the casual factors of voice disorders; and voice care and conservation. The systematic review did not found sufficient evidence to support statements that either direct or indirect or even both combined are actually effective for improving vocal functioning when measured using self-reported outcomes and when compared to no intervention. [7]

Some reports have evaluated the effectiveness of training using direct intervention techniques alone compared to no intervention. In general, direct techniques focus on the underlying physiological changes needed to improve an individual´s technique in using the vocal system. These techniques include training focused on posture, respiration, release of tension in the vocal tract, resonance and voice projection. [7]

Voice training can consist of vocal warm-up and cool-down as well as group activities regarding the psychodynamics of voice production. In order to promote vocal warm-up, facilitating sounds, body movement techniques with sounds production, overarticulation exercises, semi-occluded vocal tract exercises and chant talk exercises have been used. Direct voice training can also include warm-up, stretching, contracting, forced adduction and strengthening exercises to be practiced at home, twice per day, preferably morning and evening for a six-week period. [7].

Indirect voice training alone has been compared to no intervention. Indirect techniques concentrate on the contributory and maintenance aspects of the voice disorders (such as lack of knowledge). Indirect training can consist of providing information on the mechanics of voice production, the amount and type of voice use, vocal behaviors thought to be traumatic for the vocal cords, hydration issues, and lifestyle and diet factors that can support or interfere with a healthy voice. Patients are informed of the prevalence and impact of voice problems in teachers; basic anatomy and physiology of voice production; symptoms of voice disorders; strategies to reduce harmful vocal behaviors; managing and minimizing health factors for the development and maintenance of voice problems; and changes in the speaking environment than increase vocal efficiency and reduce vocal injuries. [7]

Lectures can be offered concerning the main factors causing vocal loading in teachers, methods available include: avoid overloading and basics of economic versus non-economic voice use. The voice training is geared towards gaining ease and endurance in voice production as well as getting rid of any poor vocal habits. The learning methods are usually introspections, discussions, voice exercises and individualized homework aimed to finding economic voice production, i.e. avoidance of excessive muscle tension of the larynx; deep breathing technique; firmness of phonation without effort; well-resonating voice quality to improve audibility; and adequate individual pitch and loudness range and variation. Patients can also receive voice hygiene lectures and in addition undergo voice massage ™ in several sessions. Voice Massage ™ consists of manipulation of voice and speech production muscles of the larynx, respiration and articulation. It also includes some vocal and respiratory exercises during manipulation. [7].

Some studies focus on direct and indirect voice training combined. Interventions consist of lectures and a practical session. The lectures concern anatomy and physiology of phonation, causes and predisposing factors to abnormal vocal fold pathology, warning symptoms of vocal fatigue, voice ergonomics (i.e. vocal hygiene, strategies to reduce vocal demand in the classroom, and changing behaviors in daily life to reduce vocal abuse), classroom acoustics, and amplification systems. Practical sessions consist of group voice therapy training: efficient respiratory behavior; laryngeal muscle relaxation; manual circumlaryngeal therapy; relaxed voicing with elimination of hard glottal attack, chewing, voicing, yawn-sigh, chant talk and pitch inflections; proper oral-nasal resonance; and developing greater oral opening [7].

Another study evaluated the effectiveness of two different programs of voice treatments on a heterogeneous group of dysphonic speakers and the stability of therapeutic progress during long term follow-up post - intervention period by using a limited multidimensional protocol of evaluation. Pathologies included vocal nodules, polyps, angiomatous polyps, Reinke's edema and hypotonic dysphonia. Patients were assigned to one of two groups, the participants in the first group received voice-therapy consisting of five phases of basic information and counseling, relaxation, breathing, emission and placement, and carryover. The total number of sessions per participant was 24 which were conducted over a period of 12 weeks. Each session lasted approximately 45 minutes. In contrast, participants included in the second group received a voice hygiene program. These patients followed guidelines for a program previously described as successful when it was used for teachers. An initial informative session lasting approximately 60 minutes was provided. The results of this study suggest that voice-therapy (direct approach) seems to be more effective than the vocal-hygiene program (indirect approach). The significantly better improvement was detected in most of the hard - dimensional variables which were used for assessing outcome, including: Aerodynamic measurements, acoustic parameters and self – rating.

Qualitative – perceptual variables including: laryngoscopy findings and spectrographic analysis also showed better outcome in patients undergoing the direct approach. The stability of these changes is usually extended during long term post - intervention follow-up period. [8]

According to another systematic revision, direct voice therapies seem to be more effective than indirect voice therapies. [9]

In studies of some specific voice therapies methods, such as manual laryngeal tension reduction and the Accent method, positive post - therapy outcomes are more frequently reported than in other studies in which therapy methodology is not clearly defined. [10]

Voice therapy approaches are often divided into three main categories: hygienic (improving behaviors than can lead to injury of the vocal folds), symptomatic (targeting treatment of abnormal voice quality in the resulting phonated voice), and physiological (optimizing voice production). These techniques have proven to be effective both in adults and in children. However, it should be pointed out that in children, the compliance of the family for modifying family's style of voice use is essential for a successful outcome. [10, 11]

CONCLUSION

Vocal nodules are the pathological result of vocal abuse and misuse. This pathology has been found predominantly in voice professionals and patients with an inadequate vocal hygiene including children. The resulting dysphonia brings consequences in psychological, socio-economic, family, and labor aspects. The best approach for tackling this disorder seems to be a multidisciplinary methodology, covering both medical and therapeutic aspects, using several therapeutic techniques including indirect and direct approaches.

An early diagnosis and treatment can prevent surgical treatment as well as consequences involving professional and personal aspects of the patient's life style.

REFERENCES

[1] Dejonckere, PH, Kob, M. Phatogenesis of vocal fold nodules: new insights from a modeling approach, *Folia Phoniatr Logop* 2009; 61: 171-179.

[2] Shah, RK. Woodnorth, H,. Glunn, A, Nuss, RC. Pediatric vocal nodules: correlation with perceptual voice analysis, *Int J Pediatr Otorhinolaryngol* 2005; 69: 903-909.

[3] Holmberg E, Hillman,R, Hammarberg, B, Sodersten, M, Doyle, P. Efficacy of a behaviorally based voice therapy protocol for vocal nodules. *Journal of Voice* 2001; 15: 395-412.

[4] Elhendi W, Santos S, Vázquez I. Effectiveness of the rehabilitator vocal treatment in patients with vocal nodules. *Acta otorrinolaringol cir cabeza cuello* 2011; 39: 175-180.

[5] Lee, EK, Son, YI. Muscle tension dysphonia in children: voice characteristics and autocome of voice therapy, *Int J Pediatr Otorhinolaryngol* 2005; 69: 911-917.

[6] Merati, AL, Keppel, K, Braun, NM, Blumin, JH, Kerschner, JE. Pediatric voice-related quality of life: findings in healthy children and in common laryngeal disorders. *Ann Otol Rhinol Laryngol* 2008; 117: 259-272.

[7] Ruotsalainen JH, Sellman J, Lehto L, Isotalo LK, Verbeek JH. Interventions for preventing voice disorders in adults. *Cochrane Database of Systematic Reviews 2007;* Issue 4. Art. No.: CD006372. DOI: 10.1002/14651858.CD006372. Pub 2.

[8] Rodríguez-Parra, M, Casado, J. Comparing voice-therapy and vocal-hygiene treatments in dysphonia using a limited multidimensional evaluation protocol. *Journal of Communication* Disorders 2011; 44: 615-630.

[9] Speyer, R. Effects of voice therapy: a systematic review. *Journal of Voice* 2008; 22: 565-580.

[10] Ozgul, AS, Muzzeyyen, C. Effects of voice therapy in school-Age Children. *Journal of Voice* 2013; 27: 787.e19-787.e25.

[11] Valadez V, Ysunza A, Ocharan. E, Garrido N, Sanchez A, Pamplona M. Voice parameters and videonasolaryngoscopy in children with vocal nodules: A longitudinal study, before and after voice therapy. *Int Journal of Pediatr Otorhinolaryngol* 2012; 76: 1361–1365.

In: Speech, Language and Voice Pathology ISBN: 978-1-63321-958-8
Editor: Pablo Antonio Ysunza

Chapter 2

Speech and Language Pathology Interventions in Critical Care: A Retrospective View

Kathleen V. Roeder*
Department of Speech and Language Pathology,
Beaumont Health System. Royal Oak, MI, US

Abstract

Speech and Language Pathology interventions in critical care purport to improve patient care and patient outcomes by addressing the risk for aspiration due to iatrogenic dysphagia related to tracheostomy tube placement, ventilator dependency and critical illness myopathy. Many Speech Pathology recommendations address NPO status, need for alternative feeding via Corpak tube and need for PEG tube placement. A retrospective analysis of 20 patients admitted to the various medical neurosurgical and surgical ICU's analyzed patients from two groups: those who were kept NPO until a Speech and Language Pathologist assessed swallow function and those who had an oral diet assigned by the medical team without an initial formal Speech Pathology swallow assessment. Among the parameters investigated were LOS in the ICU, need for re-intubation, number of NPO status days, recommendation for Corpak tube or PEG tube and discharge status with respect to oral feeding, tube feeding and modified diet.

* Contact: roederkathy@gmail.com.

Keywords: Swallowing, Dysphagia, Tracheostomy, Gastrostomy, Speech and Language Pathology

INTRODUCTION

Speech and language Pathology interventions in critical care purport to improve patient care and overall patient outcomes by addressing the risk for aspiration due to iatrogenic dysphagia from tracheostomy tube placement, vent dependency and critical illness myopathy. [1]

Many Speech Pathologists directly recommend NPO status, post suggestions for placement of a Corpak tube due to NPO status and suggest PEG tube placement. [2] Specific recommendations for oral feeding with modified diets are part of the Speech Pathology plan of care. At the conclusion of their evaluations Speech Pathologists generally decide that patients have benefitted from these recommendations. However, the medical team may conclude that patients seen by Speech Pathology receive higher numbers of recommendations for tube feedings, have longer patient stays and that the recommendations by Speech Pathology further complicate the medical course; the placement of feeding tubes can cause more complications, result in dislodged tubes and extra procedures for replacing them, complicate the discharge plan and therefore increase length of stay. [3]

PURPOSE

The purpose of this study was to compare the clinical outcome for ICU patients who were kept NPO until a swallow assessment was completed by Speech Pathology with patients who were initially given oral diets by the medical team in the absence of a formal Speech Pathology assessment.

MATERIALS AND METHODS

A retrospective analysis of 20 patients placed in the ICU between January 1, 2014 and February 28, 2014 was completed. The data collected addressed the patients' overall length of stay, the total number of procedures completed by Speech Pathology; the number of NPO days recommended by Speech

Pathology; the number of instances in which feeding tubes were recommended by Speech Pathology; the number of patients requiring re-intubation for respiratory distress, and the discharge plan specific to oral feeding recommendations.

Patients were divided into two groups. In Group 1, 10 of the patients reviewed had been NPO until seen by a Speech Pathologist. Of this first group, the medical team had determined that the patient would be best served by remaining NPO until a formal clinical swallowing assessment could be completed.

This assessment took place bedside with the actual number and type of food items presented left to the discretion of the evaluating clinician. The recommendation for an instrumental evaluation, specifically Modified Barium Swallow Study, was made by the Speech Pathologist who completed that initial clinical swallow assessment and not by another member of the medical team.

In Group 2, 10 of the patients reviewed were placed on oral feeding by the medical team and were not initially seen for a standard clinical assessment by Speech and Language Pathology. Either the rounding physician or the bedside nurse determined that the patient had a functional swallow for oral feeding. This last group of patients was eventually assessed by Speech Pathology, either for later issues potentially related to dysphagia, or for interventions related to parameters outside of swallow function, specifically dysphonia or language and cognitive dysfunction.

The patients selected retrospectively were randomly chosen from those placed in the various surgical, neurosurgical, cardiac and medical ICU's during the two month period noted above. Patient diagnoses were highly variable and included multiple trauma with traumatic brain injury, subarachnoid hemorrhage, complications associated with cardiovascular surgery, hemorrhagic CVA, craniotomy for brain tumor excision, and post-surgical respiratory failure.

All of the patients had been intubated, some of them had tracheostomy tubes at the time of evaluation; other patients were tracheostomy tube free.

RESULTS

Results of Patients with NPO Status Until Seen by Speech and Language Pathology

The Average Number of ICU Days:	9.5
The Average Number of Visits by Speech Pathology:	3.3
The Number of Patients Receiving Modified Barium Swallow Study:	3
Average Number of NPO Days After Seen By Speech Pathology:	2
Number of PEG Tube Recommendations:	0
Number of Corpak Tube Recommendations:	1
Number of Modified Diets Recommended:	7
Number of Patients Discharged on Soft or Regular Diet with Thin Liquid:	7
Number of Patients Discharged from the Hospital on Thickened Liquids:	2
Number of Patients Discharged to a Long Term Care Facility with Corpak Tube in Place:	1
Number of Re-Intubations Specific to Presumed Oropharyngeal Aspiration:	0

Results of Patients Starting Oral Feeding Before Evaluation by Speech and Language Pathology

The Average Number of ICU Days:	11.1
The Average Number of Visits by Speech Pathology:	4
The Number of Patients Receiving Modified Barium Swallow Study:	4
Average Number of NPO days after being seen by Speech Pathology:	4
Number of PEG Tube Placement Recommendations by Speech Pathology:	0
Number of Corpak Tube Recommendations:	3
Number of Modified Diets Recommended:	9
Number of Patients Discharged on Soft or Regular Diet with Thin Liquid:	6
Number of Patients Discharged to ECF with PEG Tube in Place:	1
Number of Patients Discharged to ECF with Corpak tube in Place:	0
Number of Re-intubations Specific to Presumed Oropharyngeal Aspiration:	2

Discussion

The ten patients In Group 1, who were NPO until seen by Speech Pathology for a formal clinical swallow assessment, had no instances of oropharyngeal aspiration. Two out of the second group of 10 patients developed increased respiratory distress and required re-intubation. While it is difficult to draw a direct correlation between increased respiratory distress and oropharyngeal aspiration, the medical team deemed aspiration a consideration to be resolved by a Speech Pathology evaluation. [4] On completion of a Modified Barium Swallow, both of these patients were found to have aspiration of at least one food and one liquid consistency. Unresolved questions include the possibility that the overall medical course was more complicated and that dysphagia was therefore a later consequence of those complications. It is certainly possible that the need for repeated intubation and prolonged NPO status as a result of intubation contributed to the MBS findings and that prior to re-intubation swallow function had been better. Also under consideration is the possibility that those two patients had less stable respiratory status than the others and developed increased risk for aspiration simply due to the added labor of trying to coordinate respiration with swallow initiation. [5] However, with any of those considerations in mind, a formal clinical swallow evaluation might have concluded that those two patients would be best served by short term NPO status while respiratory function stabilized.

With the exception of one patient who was seen for a language assessment post hemorrhagic stroke all of the patients in Group 2 developed some complication related to respiratory function that increased the medical team's concern for underlying dysphagia and associated aspiration as a potential factor in the change in respiratory status. Of the 10 patients in Group 2 who eventually received a consultation for Speech Pathology all but one of them were found to have dysphagia requiring at least a modified diet. Were the modified diets warranted? Should the patients have had Modified Barium Swallow Studies? Were those studies simply added cost? Was respiratory distress going to occur whether or not Speech Pathology was involved? Were the changes in respiration really associated with swallow dysfunction or were those events specific to other medical issues? While it is not within the scope of this simple retrospective analysis to determine whether the presence of Speech Pathology would have reduced the risks for increasing respiratory distress or prevented the need for re-intubation, these are important questions for both Speech Pathologists and the primary medical team. [6] The relative cost versus the relative gain from a formal swallow assessment for the ICU patient who develops increased respiratory compromise is a quality and safety issue for the patient and the critical care team.

So, if we cannot yet answer the questions posed above, what conclusions can be drawn from the information provided?

CONCLUSION

The conclusions we can draw from this small sample of ICU patients over a two month period are these:

1. No PEG tubes were recommended by Speech Pathology in either group.
2. 10% of patients in Group 1 received a suggestion for Corpak tube placement while 30% of patients in Group 2 received a suggestion for Corpak tube placement.
3. 30% of patients in the first group had Modified Barium Swallows Studies while 40% of patients in the second group had Modified Barium Swallow Studies.
4. No patients in the first group developed respiratory distress complicating length of stay or requiring re-intubation.
5. 20% of patients in the second group developed respiratory distress with aspiration a consideration but undetermined as a final etiology.
6. The total number of procedures completed by Speech Pathology was three for Group 1, and four for Group 2.
7. Group 2 had an increased number of NPO days.
8. Respiratory distress is often multifactorial and may not result specifically from aspiration, but aspiration does surface as a potential etiology when respiratory distress develops during a hospitalization.
9. Once the issue of respiratory distress and re-intubation surfaced, more procedures and less reliance on clinical bedside swallow evaluation also surfaced.
10. There was increased reliance on use of MBSS once patients had attempted oral feeding and then developed respiratory distress.

IMPLICATIONS FOR SPEECH PATHOLOGY AND FOR THE CRITICAL CARE TEAM

The formal clinical swallow evaluation can be an effective, timely and cost effective strategy for the ICU patient. A Modified Barium Swallow Study is not always needed before starting an oral diet. The best course of action in the critically ill patient who is increasingly challenged by weak breath support might well be to instate NPO status or limit po intake to compensate for generalized weakness, poor endurance and associated weak breath support until respiratory function stabilizes. [7]

While daily intervention from Speech Pathology is not easily proved cost effective in the ICU, an initial clinical evaluation and a limited number of follow up visits can be cost effective by forwarding patient progress through safe oral feeding without incurring the significant cost associated with numerous procedures. While the double blind study is the gold standard for accurate determination of outcomes, most physicians are reluctant to withhold services from one patient while providing them to another patient. Therefore, an ongoing data collection might well be an important starting point for determining patient outcomes. Most importantly, this retrospective analysis will result in the collection of data in our department from the point forward in order to identify the relative cost and safety benefit to the ICU patient from our service, as well as to identify potential costs and complications associated with Speech Pathology recommendations.

REFERENCES

[1] Romero, CM MD; Marambia, A, MD; Larrondo, J, MD, Walker, K, MD; Lira, MT, RN; Tobar, E, MD; Cornejo, R, MD; Ruiz, M, MD: Swallowing dysfunction in nonneurologic critically ill patients who require percutaneous dilatational tracheostomy: *Chest* 2010 137(6):1278-1282.

[2] Janes SE, Price CS, Khan S. Percutaneous endoscopic gastrostomy: mortality trends and risk factors. *J. Postgrad Med* 2005:51 23-29.

[3] Halloran O, Grecu B, Sinha A. Methods and Complications of Nasoenteral Intubation. *JPEN J. Parenteral Enteral Nutr* 2011; 35(1):61-66.

[4] Krishnan, Raghavendran. MD; Nemzek, Jean DVM, MS; Napolitano, Lena MD; Knight, Paul, MD, PhD. *Aspiration-Induced lung injury: Critical Care Med.* Apr 2011:39(4):818-826.

[5] Martin-Harris B, Brodsky MB, Price CC, Michel Y, Walters B: (2oo3) Temporal coordination of pharyngeal and laryngeal dynamics with breathing during swallowing: Single liquid swallows: *JApp Physiology.* 94, 1735-1743.

[6] Moraes, DP, Sassi FC, Mangilli, LD, Zilberstein, B, Furquim de Andrade, C R: *Clinical prognostic indicators of dysphagia following prolonged orotracheal intubation in ICU patients:* Critical Care 2013.

[7] Yarborough M. Why physicians must not give food and water to every patient *JFam Pract* 1989; 683-684.

In: Speech, Language and Voice Pathology ISBN: 978-1-63321-958-8
Editor: Pablo Antonio Ysunza

Chapter 3

SPEECH SOUND DISORDERS PROTOCOL GUIDE FOR SPEECH AND LANGUAGE PATHOLOGISTS

Marisa Lousada[1*] and Margarida Ramalho[2†]
[1]School of Health Sciences (ESSUA), University of Aveiro, Aveiro and Center for Health Technology and Services Research (CINTESIS), Porto, Portugal
[2]School of Health Sciences, Polytechnic Institute of Setúbal (IPS), Setúbal, Portugal

ABSTRACT

Children with speech sound disorders (SSD) dominate the caseloads of many speech and language pathologists (SLPs) and form a heterogeneous group [1,2]. The clinical practice with children with SSD involves several methods and theoretical assumptions. Different procedures should be considered in the assessment of children with SSD, e.g., case history, single word test, stimulability, oral motor-speech, phonological analysis (linear and non-linear), phonological awareness, syllable/ word shapes, intelligibility [3]. Also, a large number of intervention approaches are available for children with SSD [4,5], for example, minimal opposition contrast therapy [6], traditional articulation

* E-mail: marisalousada@ua.pt.
† E-mail: amargaridamcramalho@gmail.com.

therapy [7], core vocabulary [8], cycles approach [9], phonological awareness [10]. It has also been suggested that some intervention approaches are more effective for some SSD subgroups [11–14].

More recently SLPs are also encouraged to use the International Classification of Functioning, Disability and Health (ICF) [WHO 15], or the International Classification of Functioning, Disability and Health Children and Youth Version (ICF-CY) [WHO 16] in order to contemplate not only the speech disorders (body structures/ functions) but also its impact in person's activities and participation and the contextual factors (environmental and personal) that affect communication. As professional associations suggests [ASHA 17,RCSLT 18,CASLPA 19] ICF can help SLPs using a common terminology system by adaptation of many classifications that are already in use.

Since clinicians have limited time and access to analyze all of the relevant studies about assessment and intervention for children with SSD and incorporate ICF in their clinical practice, we intend with this chapter to guide them to implement best practice for children with SSD in terms of clinical process (since case history to intervention outcomes) and include ICF terminology in all process. Specifically we will present the *SSD protocol guide for SLPs.*

Keywords: Speech sound disorders, assessment, intervention, ICF

INTRODUCTION

Speech sound disorders (SSD) are the most common diagnosis made by speech and language pathologists (SLPs) working with preschool and school aged children [1,2]. Some children have a speech sound disorder that is secondary to conditions such as hearing impairment, cognitive impairment or cleft lip and/or palate but for the majority the cause is unknown [2]. In this chapter we will focus on SSD of unknown origin.

Research has showed that SSD form a heterogeneous group, thus several procedures should be used in the assessment and intervention with these children. This chapter will present a proposal for the *SSD protocol guide for SLPs.* This guide provides current information about the terminology, assessment, and intervention and the use of the International Classification of Functioning, Disability and Health (ICF) [WHO 15], and the International Classification of Functioning, Disability and Health Children and Youth Version (ICF-CY) [WHO 16] in these disorders.

SSD PROTOCOL GUIDE FOR SLPS

The International Classification of Functioning, Disability and Health (ICF) is one of the World Heath Organization (WHO) frameworks. The previous classification (International Classification of Impairments, Disabilities and Handicaps (ICIDH), published in 1980 focused in the disease, but ICF changes this paradigm, into bio psychosocial paradigm giving much importance to individual health and functioning.

According to Reed et al. [20] the ICF classification allows the documentation of the impact of health conditions on human functioning from the biological, individual and societal perspectives. Thus, ICF classification is very useful for SLP, since communication disorders can implicate body structures and functions and has consequences in person's activities and participation.

Also, ICF integrate contextual factors (environmental and personal factors). In environmental factors it is important to consider many physical, social and attitudinal environment which people live and conduct their lives [WHO 16]. For example, the SLP himself (e355 health professionals) can be considered as a facilitator or a barrier. When SLP is a facilitator he or she helps child with SSD, improving functionality in child's most important contexts (e.g. family routines, kindergarten, school and other social events). ICF conceptualizes functioning and disability as a dynamic interaction between a person's health condition and their Contextual Factors [WHO 15] (see Figure 1).

Several of international professional associations recommend the use of ICF in SLPs clinical practice aiming clinical goals, professional interest and scientific research in communication disorders. ASHA [21] suggests that SLPs apply ICF in all intervention domains, such as prevention, assessment, intervention and scientific study of communication and swallowing disorders. In the same way, CASLPA [19] encourages the development of outcome measures considering ICF and the ICF-CY classifications.

The Resource Manual for Commissioning and Planning Services for SLCN, published by Royal College of Speech and Language Therapists [22] describes the impact level that speech sound disorders can have in children's system, for each ICF dimensions. The impairment can involve sound production, phonological awareness, phonological processing, phonological template, segmentation skills, mental representation of words in the lexicon and prosody. In the same way, activity can be affected as well, in areas like intelligibility of speech, reading and writing skills. Once reduced, communication skills can affect self-esteem, self-identity, relationships, educational and work attainment [RCSLT, 22].

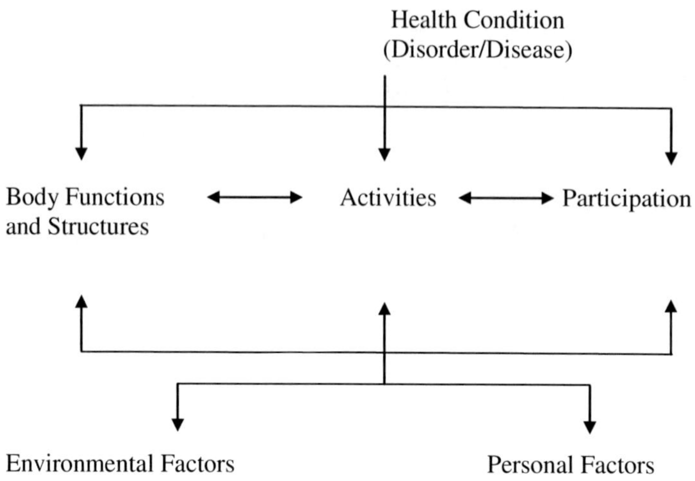

Figure 1. Representation of the *International Classification of Functioning, Disability and Health* (ICF) [WHO 15].

One of the principal aims is to provide an interdisciplinary consensual terminology for health professionals by using a standard language and framework. However, in SSD area there are some issues with the terminology used and the underlying problems for diagnosis description, which could have a considerable impact in assessment and intervention. These particular aspects are discussed in the following sections.

Body Functions

McCormack and Worral [23] reported the ICF Body Functions related to speech-language pathology. The application of ICF codes to SSD usually contemplates primarily *articulation functions* (b320). Other codes are also referred (*mental functions of sequencing complex movements* – b176 and *fluency and rhythm of speech functions* – b 330) to describe SSD of unknown origin.

In some SSD sub-groups, where linguistic competence is affected (e.g. phonology), it´s not common the use of language related codes in the assessment/analysis and intervention [23, 24].

In the authors' perspective, phonology is one of the linguistic domains, so *mental functions of language* (b167) should be used to classify some SSD sub-groups (phonological delay, consistent atypical phonological disorder, inconsistent phonological disorder and CAS/DVD) (see table 1).

Table 1. SSD sub-groups proposed by Dodd [25] and possible related ICF codes

Dodd's five subgroups	Codes usually used to classify SSD [24]	Proposal considering phonology as a linguistic process*
Articulation disorder	b320	b320
Phonological delay	b320	b167 b320
Consistent atypical phonological disorder	b320	b167 b320
Inconsistent phonological disorder	b320	b167 b320
Childhood apraxia of speech (CAS)/ Developmental verbal dyspraxia (DVD)	b320	b176 b320 b167

* Codes are hierarchy organised by level of impact.

Activity and Participation

The Activities and Participation component of the ICF describes the human functioning from the individual to a societal perspective. So the *activity* is referred to ''the execution of a task or action by an individual'' - individual perspective. *Participation* include ''involvement in a life situation'' - societal perspective [WHO, 16].

Regarding the third chapter of ICF, the *Activity and Participation component* focuses on *Communication* describing it in terms of type of message received or produced (*communicating - receiving* (d310-d329) and *communicating - producing* - d330-d349), whether it is non-verbal or verbal (modality) and in terms of the modality the person uses to communicate like body gestures and drawings. However, communication activity and participation is also mentioned in other chapters like *learning and applied knowledge* or *interpersonal interactions and relationships* [26].

CONTEXTUAL FACTORS

The second part of ICF is related to Contextual Factors that ‘‘represent the complete background of an individual’s life and living’’ (WHO, 2001, p. 16) and contain two components - Environmental Factors and Personal Factors. Environmental Factors include all aspects of the external world of an individual’s life that may have an impact on his or her functioning. Personal Factors comprise ‘‘features of the individual that are not part of the health condition’’ such as gender, age, and coping styles (WHO, 2001, p. 17).

CLINICAL HISTORY

Case history questions allow SLPs to obtain background information about the child to a better understanding of the problem and to plan treatment. This section will focus on specific questions for SSD and its relation to ICF.

The aim of the questions about communication history is to determine if the child has evidenced delay in the attainment of principal language milestones [27]. Questions about birth and medical history are included to know if any medical factors could have influenced communication development, to conclude if the child has a SSD secondary to other condition (e.g., hearing impairment – b230 hearing functions) or an SSD of unknown origin.

When SLP do the child's clinical history, he or she should also consider environmental factors like *support and relationships* (e3), such as *immediate family* (e310) or *friends* (e320), or *attitudes* (e4) (e.g. *individual attitudes of immediately family members* (e410). Thus, social history will help to determine if a child has had opportunities to communicate and if the environment is sufficiently rich to foster adequate communication development [27]. It is also important to know for example if the caregivers are always correcting speech errors because too much correction can have a negative impact (e.g., frustration). It is essential to balance between correcting errors, praising success and letting some errors pass [28]. It is very important to know about the environmental factors and assess their impact on SSD and intervention process.

Finally, the aim in obtaining an education history is to know if a child has received school services (e.g. regular class at school (e585)) and also if he or she received any special services (special education and training services (e5853)) [27].

Assessment

Different procedures should be take into account in the assessment of children with SSD, specifically, case history, single word test, stimulability, oral motor-speech, phonological analysis (linear and non-linear), phonological awareness, syllable/ word shapes, intelligibility [3]. McLeod and Threats [24] presented a list of assessments and analysis of SSD children's and the ICF-CY codes usually associated: *auditory perception* (b1560), *fluency and rhythm of speech functions* (b330), *mental function of sequencing complex movements* (b176), *articulation function* (b320) (body functions); *structure of the mouth* (s320) (body structures); *learning to read* (d140), *communication* (d3), *interpersonal interactions and relationships* (d7), *major life areas* (d8), *community, social and civic life* (d9) (activity and participation).

Considering that SSD covers different underlying problems (e.g., motoric, phonological) in the present proposal other codes should be added to a better description of the assessment/analysis used. For example when the SLPs use a phonological analysis in a child with a phonological delay or disorder, the code *mental functions of language* (b167) seems to help in a better representation of the type of SSD, because in a phonological perspective phonology is part of language.

Mental functions of language refer to "specific mental functions of recognizing and using signs, symbols and other components of a language" (WHO, 2007, 58) and phonology is one of the language components. It is important to dissociate phonetics (articulation based problems) from phonology (linguistically-based problems) [29,30]. Thus, in a way to improve evidence-based practice, this underlying concept should be present in the assessment and intervention with children with phonologically based SSD.

INTERVENTION APPROACHES FOR CHILDREN WITH SSD

At the moment different intervention approaches are used for children with SSD [4,5], e.g. minimal opposition contrast therapy [6], traditional articulation therapy [7], core vocabulary [8], cycles approach [9], and phonological awareness [10].

Table 2. Comparison of the Impairment Scale proposed by Enderby at al (2006, p. 90) and ICF Body Functions and Structures extent or magnitude scale of an impairment (WHO, 2001) for phonologically based SSD

Enderby et al. (2006)	ICF
Impairment	**Body Functions and Structures**
0 Totally limited sound system; uses no recognisable consonants.	xxx.4 **Complete** impairment (total,…) 96-100%
1 Speech system restricted; uses a few recognisable sounds including some consonants.	xxx.3 **Severe** impairment (high, extreme,…) 50-95
2 Good use of consonants and vowels at single word level but poor transfer of sounds into sentences. May have 25% to 50% suppression of inappropriate processes.	xxx.2 **Moderate** impairment (medium, fair,...) 25-49 %
3 Capable of clear speech when thinking about it and prompted, but clarity deteriorates in spontaneous speech. May have 50% to 75% suppression of inappropriate processes.	
4 Persistent minor immaturities; may have typical processes at a later age or one atypical process.	xxx.1 **Mild** impairment (slight, low,…) 5-24 %
5 Age-appropriate speech	xxx. 0 No impairment (none, absent, negligible,…) 0-4 %
	xxx.8 not specified
	xxx.9 not applicable

Intervention studies indicated that some intervention approaches are more effective for some SSD subgroups, for example phonological therapy was found to be more effective than articulation therapy for children with phonologically based SSD [13,14]. Also, according to Dodd and colleagues [11,12] children with inconsistent phonological disorder received most benefit from the core vocabulary approach and children with consistent speech disorder improved more with phonological contrast therapy.

Concerning outcome measures, studies typically provide speech severity indices, for example, percentage of occurrence of phonological processes and percentage of consonant correct (PCC) score [4]. However, intelligibility should also be used as an outcome measure as with this measure we can analyse the impact of the disorder in the activity and participation level (see Tables 2 and 3).

In Table 4 it is proposed a checklist of ICF codes for SSD, which contains the possible codes (body functions and structures, activity and participation, environmental factors) to be used along the clinical process i.e. since clinical history to intervention. Despite some of the codes are not essential (e.g., structure of mouth) in SSD of unknown origin, we also include it because it is important in a way to establish the differential diagnosis between a primary and a secondary SSD.

Table 3. Comparison Activity and Participation scales of ICF (WHO, 2001) and Enderby at al (2006, p. 90) for phonologically based SSD

Enderby et al. (2006)		**ICF**
Activity	**Participation**	**Activity and Participation**
0 Completely unintelligible to familiar and non-familiar listeners.	**0** Unable to fulfil any social/educational/family role. Not involved in decision-making/no autonomy/ no control over environment, no social integration.	xxx.4 **Complete** difficulty (total,…) 96-100%
1 Partly intelligible to familiar listeners in known context; communication partner bears the burden of the responsibility.	**1** Low self-confidence/poor self-esteem/limited social integration/socially isolated/contributes to some basic and limited decisions. Cannot achieve potential in any situation.	xxx.3 **Severe** difficulty (high, extreme,…) 50-95

Table 3. (Continued)

Enderby et al. (2006)		**ICF**
Activity	**Participation**	**Activity and Participation**
2 Intelligible to familiar listeners in context; partly intelligible in context with non-familiar listeners; single words clear, connected speech poor.	**2** Some self-confidence/some social integration/makes some decisions and influences control in familiar situations.	xxx.2 **Moderate** difficulty (medium, fair,...) 25-49 %
3 Usually intelligible to familiar listeners in and out of context; variable intelligibility in context with non-familiar listeners; free, spontaneous speech often unintelligible.	**3** Some self-confidence; autonomy emerging. Makes decisions and has control of some aspects of life. Able to achieve some limited social integration/educational activities. Diffident over control over life. Needs encouragement to achieve potential.	
4 Minor problems but intelligible to everyone; occasionally loses intelligibility at times, for example when excited or speaking against noise, etc.	**4** Mostly confident; occasional difficulties integrating or in fulfilling social/role activity. Participating in all appropriate decisions. May have difficulty in achieving potential in some situations occasionally.	xxx.1 **Mild** difficulty (slight, low,…) 5-24 %
5 Intelligible at age-appropriate level to familiar listeners and non-familiar listeners.	**5** Achieving potential. Autonomous and unrestricted. Able to fulfil social, educational and family role.	xxx. 0 **No** difficulty (none, absent, negligible,…) 0-4 %
		xxx.8 not specified
		xxx.9 not applicable

Table 4. Checklist – ICF codes for SSD

Checklist - ICF codes for SSD (WHO, 2001; WHO, 2007)

Name: ____

Date: ___/____/_______ Diagnose:
____

Speech and Language Pathologist: ____
Observations:

____

____

____

	Qualifiers						
Body structures	0	1	2	3	4	8	9
Chapter 3 - Structures involved in voice and speech							
s310 Structure of nose							
s320 Structure of mouth							
Chapter 7 - Structures related to movement							
s710 Structure of head and neck region							
Other codes							
Body functions	0	1	2	3	4	8	9
Specific mental functions							
b156 Perceptual functions							
b1560 Auditory perception							
b 167 Mental functions of language							
b16708 Reception of language, other specified							
b16718 Expression of language, other specified							

Table 4. (Continued)

b176 Mental function of sequencing complex movements							
Voice and speech functions							
b320 Articulation functions							
b330 Fluency and rhythm of speech functions							
b3300 Fluency of speech							
b3301 Rhythm of speech							
b3302 Speed of speech							
b3303 Melody of speech							
Other codes							
Activity and Participation	0	1	2	3	4	8	9
Chapter 1 - Learning and applying knowledge							
Basic learning (d130-d159)							
Applying knowledge (d160-d179)							
Chapter 3 - Communication							
Communicating - receiving (d310-d329)							
Communicating - producing (d330-d349)							
Conversation and use of communication devices and techniques (d350-d369)							
Chapter 7 - Interpersonal interaction and relationships							
General interpersonal interaction (d710-d729)							
Particular interpersonal relationships (d730-d739)							
Chapter 8 - Major life areas							
Education (d810-d839)							
Chapter 9 -Community, social and civic life							

d920- Recreation and leisure							
Other codes							
Environmental factors	0	1	2	3	4	8	9
Chapter 1 - Products and technology							
e115 Products and technology for personal use in daily living							
e125 Products and technology for communication							
Chapter 3 - Support and relationships							
e310 Immediate family							
e315 Extended family							
e320 Friends							
e325 Acquintances, peers, colleagues, neighbours and community members							
e330 People in positions of authority							
e355 Health professionals (SLP and others)							
e360 Other professionals							
Chapter 4 - Attitudes							
e410 Individual attitudes of immediate family members							
e415 Individual attitudes of extended family members							
e420 Individual attitudes of friends							
e425 Individual attitudes of acquintances, peers, colleagues, neighbours and community members							
e450 Individual attitudes of health professionals							
e455 Individual attitudes of other professionals							
Chapter 5 - Services, systems and policies							
e580 Health services, systems and policies							
e585 Education and training services, systems and policies							

Conclusion

Considering that ICF framework is recommended for SLPs clinical practice, the main goal with this chapter was to highlight not only the disorder but also the interaction between body structure and functions and environmental factors (positive - facilitators or negative - barriers) that have an impact on impairment and functioning levels. Thus, it is important to analyse all these components to an holistically assessment of SSD children.

In the first approaches about the use of ICF related to SLPs, some authors have been presented ICF codes that could be used to describe SSD children. However, the main code commonly used for all SSD is *articulation functions*. With the presented proposal we intend to describe phonologically based SSD using ICF codes (e.g., mental functions of language) considering the underlying phonological deficit since phonology is a language domain.

Finally it was proposed a checklist that is useful for SLPs during all the clinical process, with relevant codes that could describe children with SSD. The SLPs usually obtain information during clinical history, assessment, intervention and analyses of the efficacy and efficiency of treatment. The ICF can help the clinician in all these stages and also contribute to measure intervention outcomes.

References

[1] McLeod S, Harrison L. Epidemiology of Speech and Language Impairment in a Nationally Representative Sample of 4- to 5-Year-Old Children. *J Speech, Lang Hear Res.* 2009;52:1213–29.

[2] Waring R, Knight R. How should children with speech sound disorders be classified? A review and critical evaluation of current classification systems. *Int J Lang Commun Disord.* 2013;48(1):25–40.

[3] Skahan S, Watson M, Lof GL. Speech-language pathologists' assessment practices for children with suspected speech sound disorders: results of a national survey. *Am J Speech - Lang Pathol.* 2007;16:246–59.

[4] Baker E, McLeod S. Evidence-Based Practice for Children With Speech Sound Disorders: Part 1 Narrative Review. *Lang Speech Hear Serv Sch.* 2011;42:102–39.

[5] Joffe V, Pring T. Children with phonological problems: a survey of clinical practice. *Int J Lang Commun Disord.* 2008;43(2):154–64.

[6] Weiner F. Treatment of phonological disability using the method of meaningful contrast: Two case studies. *J Speech Hear Disord.* 1981;46:97–103.

[7] Van Riper C, Emerick L. *Speech correction: An introduction to speech pathology and audiology.* 7th ed. Englewood Cliffs: Prentice-Hall; 1984.

[8] Dodd B, Iacono T. Phonological disorders in children: changes in phonological process use during treatment. *Br J Disord Commun.* 1989;24:333–51.

[9] Hodson B, Paden E. *Targeting intelligible speech: A phonological approach to remediation.* San Diego: College-Hill Press; 1991.

[10] Gillon GT. The efficacy of phonological awareness intervention for children with spoken language impairment. *Lang Speech Hear Serv Sch.* 2000;31:126–41.

[11] Crosbie S, Holm A, Dodd B. Intervention for children with severe speech disorder: A comparison of two approaches. *Int J Lang Commun Disord.* 2005;40(4):467–91.

[12] Dodd B, Bradford A. A comparison of three therapy methods for children with different types of developmental phonological disorders. *Int J Lang Commun Disord.* 2000;35(2):189–209.

[13] Lousada M, Jesus LMT, Capelas S, Margaça C, Simões D, Valente AR, et al. Phonological and articulation treatment approaches in Portuguese children with speech and language impairments: a randomised controlled intervention study. *Int J Lang Commun Disord.* 2013;48(2):172–87.

[14] Lousada M, Jesus LMT, Hall A, Joffe V. Intelligibility as a clinical outcome measure following intervention with children with phonologically-based speech sound disorders. *Int J Lang Commun Disord.* 2014;In press.

[15] World Health Organization. *International Classification of Functioning, Disability and Health (ICF).* Geneva: WHO; 2001.

[16] World Health Organization. *International Classification of Functioning, Disability and Health Children and Youth Version (ICF-CY).* Geneva: WHO; 2007.

[17] American Speech-Language-Hearing Association. *Preferred Practice Patterns for the Profession of Speech-Language Pathology* [Preferred Practice Patterns] [Internet]. 2004. Available from: www.asha.org/policy.

[18] Royal College of Speech & Language Therapists. *Clinical Guidelines.* UK: Royal College of Speech & Language Therapists; 2009.

[19] CASLPA. *Position Statement on Outcomes Measures.* CASLPA; 2010.

[20] Reed GM, Lux JB, Bufka LF, Trask C, Peterson DB, Stark S, et al. Operationalizing the international classification of functioning, *Disability and Health in clinical settings. Rehabil Psychol.* 2005;50:122–31.

[21] American Speech-Language-Hearing Association. *Scope of Practice in Speech-Language Pathology* [Scope of Practice]. 2007.

[22] Royal College of Speech and Language Therapists. *RCSLT resource manual for commissioning and planning services for SLCN: Speech and language impairment.* RCSLT; 2009.

[23] McCormack J, Worrall LE. The ICF Body Functions and Structures related to speech-language pathology. *Int J Speech Lang Pathol.* 2008;10(1):9–17.

[24] McLeod S, Threats TT. The ICF-CY and children with communication disabilities. *Int J Speech Lang Pathol.* 2008;10:92–109.

[25] Dodd B. *Differential diagnosis and treatment of children with speech disorder.* 2nd ed. London: Whurr; 2005.

[26] O'Halloran R, Larkins B. The ICF Activities and Participation related to speech-language pathology. *Int J Speech Lang Pathol.* 2008;10(1):18–26.

[27] Bleile KM. *Manual of articulation and phonological disorders: Infance through adulthood.* 2nd ed. San Diego: Singular; 2004.

[28] Bowen C. *Developmental phonological disorders. A practical guide for families and teachers.* Melbourne: ACER Press; 1998.

[29] Baker E. Management of speech impairment in children: The journey so far and the road ahead. *Adv Speech-Language Pathol.* 2006;8(3):156–63.

[30] Grunwell P. Developmental phonological disorders: Order in disorder. In: Hodson BW, Edwards ML, editors. *Perspectives in applied phonology.* Gaithersburg, MD: Aspen; 1997. p. 61–104.

In: Speech, Language and Voice Pathology ISBN: 978-1-63321-958-8
Editor: Pablo Antonio Ysunza

Chapter 4

A Play Toolkit Used in Early Language Intervention

Kristine Rutkowski*

Department of Speech and Language Pathology,
Beaumont Health System, Royal Oak, MI, US

Abstract

Special educators often promote young children's pretend play abilities with play intervention methods because of the observed relationship between play skills and cognitive, social, and language development [1]. In a 1993 study, teachers reported that approximately 75% of children with language disorders need assistance with social play skills [2]. However, in his 1997 review of research on the symbolic play skills of children with language disabilities, M. W. Casby discovered play abilities not to be very lacking in these children [3]. Most importantly, their capabilities for using symbolic ideas in play may be similar to those of children without language disabilities, revealing "a symbolic *performance* deficit more so than a symbolic *competence* deficit. In pretend play, difficulties with language consistently get in the way of making play themes and roles explicit. Similarly, Guralnik [4] found that children with mild language disabilities tend to progress like their peers in terms of play, steadily transitioning from solitary to parallel to social play, for example, but simply taking longer to do so.

* krutkowski@beaumont.edu

There is a growing body of evidence supporting the role not only of language proficiency in pretend play but also of pretend play in the acquisition of language [5]. Specifically, the use of a variety of props and objects, combining multiple roles and themes, and creating pretend scenarios provide the best opportunities for fostering language growth. Using clearly defined, measurable language goals, the speech-language pathologist (SLP) can promote language growth by working through a pretend play developmental hierarchy. Initially, realistic props not only expand vocabulary of common objects and their functions but also help children maintain their roles and remember their play scenario while acting out activities of daily living. As pretend play advances, props become more symbolic, often taking on more than one function during play (e.g., a box used as a boat can be flipped over to be used as a cave). The SLP progressively introduces these open-ended and multi-functional items as a child's linguistic structures emerge and evolve so as to establish their relationships. Eventually, children will learn to make their own props (e.g., play dough can be shaped into a pizza) [6]. This chapter offers the SLP a play toolkit that implements a hierarchy of pretend play techniques to advance the linguistic competence of language-delayed preschoolers.

Keywords: Early intervention, play, language

INTRODUCTION

As a natural activity of early childhood, play has great relevance in the field of pediatric language delays and disorders. This chapter presents a review of literature regarding the importance of play in language development and how play is used in early language intervention.

In 1969, Piaget and Inhelder [7] proposed that, as cognition is a necessity for language acquisition, so is language part of the underlying framework for human mental representational abilities. Furthermore, symbolic play is a surface manifestation of cognitive ability [7]. Therefore, development in symbolic play must parallel development in language, as each depends on the advancement of the other, for they belong to one underlying system of mental representational capacity.

The homologue model proposed by Bates [8] also supports and explains the high correlation between symbolic play and language. This model confirmed that language and cognition both developed as stems of an underlying system of cognitive operation. Therefore, child's play skills should correlate with his or her language development. The model also advocated that language development assists the development of symbolic play skills. Therefore, the two should have a direct correlation, and symbolic play development can be attributed to the language learning process.

Lifter and Bloom [9] found that advances in play and increases in receptive and expressive language emerge in concert with each other. For example, the emergence of constructing relationships between objects in play coincided with the emergence of first words. In addition, the vocabulary spurt occurred when children were learning specific relations between objects in play, such as using soap to give their doll a bath. They also found that these developments occurred simultaneously despite the variability in chronological ages the children reached these developmental achievements. Developmental advances between play and language have also been found in other studies [10, 11].

Piaget helped us to understand the relationship and connection between play and language from the child's view. "The child does not, in the first instance, communicate with his fellow beings in order to share thoughts and reflections; he does so in order to play" [12]. It is clear to all who witness children at play that they find it rewarding and motivating. Piaget [12] first divided the sequence of children's play development into three broad categories: practice play, symbolic play, and play with rules.

Normal Development of Play and Language

Much can be revealed about the developmental status of an infant, toddler, or young child through the observation, assessment, and evaluation of his or her play. A number of professionals have noted that play is a developmental domain that is critical to early language intervention [13-15]. In fact, the development of play demonstrates a strong relationship with the constructs of the sensorimotor and preoperational periods of cognitive development [16-18]. The SLP must be an expert in aspects of play. Play activities, behaviors, and interactions are very often some of the only performances available for observation of infants, toddlers, and children suspected of having a developmental delay. Thus, play in and of itself can be the basis of a valuable developmental assessment and intervention strategy. Rossetti [13] suggested that eliciting, observing, and describing the play of infants will give the clinician the direction needed for intervention efforts.

The early play behavior of infants and toddlers is reflective of early cognitive development. For example, the early levels of sensorimotor–exploratory play and nonfunctional relational play are reflective of the early stages of sensorimotor development, whereas later forms of play, such as functional–conventional and symbolic, indicate later stages of sensorimotor development as well as early aspects of preoperational development [14]. Some researchers believe that symbolic play is an early demonstration of young children's developing mental representation and symbolic capacity and functioning [10,12]. A number of investigators have explored the developmental relationship between symbolic play and language [16-18]. The general consensus of this line of inquiry has been that early language development and symbolic play are closely correlated. Children diagnosed with specific language impairment have been researched extensively in regard to play and have consistently been found to have delays in symbolic play [19,20]. One consensus finding has been that the younger a child with developmental disabilities is, the more likely he or she is to demonstrate difficulties in play, particularly symbolic play.

The development of communication should be assessed from birth onward as infants achieve cognitive milestones that prepare them for language. Before infants are verbal, they learn to think about means and ends. For example, they may learn to pull a cloth to retrieve a toy. They also watch their caregivers and learn. An infant may copy a caregiver's actions hours after having observed the behavior. Copying an action after a delay requires the construction, storage, and retrieval of mental symbols. These cognitive achievements reflect symbolic thought and help prepare infants to use words to communicate. Observation of infant play can help determine if they are using means and ends as well as deferred imitation behaviors within the expected time frame of development.

Infants become involved in social interaction long before they begin using words. By the end of seven months, many infants are able to turn their heads when hearing their name, smile back at another person and enjoy social play such as peek-a-boo. Joint attention and shared reference are crucial social skills that develop between nine and twelve months of age. These behaviors refer to an infant's use of communicative intent, such as smiles and gestures, to gain attention of others. It is common for an infant to repair a failed communication by trying another strategy, such as squealing or crying to gain social attention. Gestures such as pointing, smiling and gaze direction are precursors to verbal language. The use of pointing is particularly important to guide the attention of others toward objects and events. Questionnaires and checklists for parents, such as the Modified Checklist for Autism in Toddlers-Revised (M-CHAT-R) [20] and the MacArthur-Bates Communicative Development Inventories [21], are important sources of information about an infant's gestural expression. When observations suggest delayed development, referral to a developmental pediatrician is recommended.

Some children may possess functional play skills, such as pushing a toy train around a track, but will have difficulty with symbolic play and play that involves joint engagement with others [22, 23]. The emergence of symbolic play is considered an important precursor to language development [15]. During the first year of life, sensorimotor, or practice, play emerges with the child manipulating objects (e.g., mouthing, holding, banging, dropping, etc.). At approximately twelve months, the child begins to combine objects in relational play (e.g., stacking, nesting, building a tower of two blocks). Functional play (e.g., rolling or throwing a ball, drinking from a cup) also begins to occur in a child's second year. This is followed by symbolic, or make-believe, play. Symbolic play may be self-directed, such as pretending to drink from a cup, or other-directed, such as pretending to give the doll a drink. Self-directed play begins before other-directed play.

Methods

Developmental Assessment of Play

The preceding has concerned the development of early cognition, play and language. This information is significant to speech-language pathologists involved in early intervention. This section presents a criterion-referenced, descriptive, and developmentally-based protocol for the dynamic observation and assessment of the play behavior of infants, toddlers, and young children. This protocol was developed from the wide array of studies that show the high level of validity and reliability of such measurement of play [24]. The assessment of play behavior must take place in a comfortable environment for the child and should feel as natural as possible. Present should be the speech-language pathologist, the child, and a parent or caregiver in the child's daily life. Symbolic play assessment provides the child objects with the potential to be transformed in play, that is, capable of standing in or substituting for other objects [25, 26]. An assortment of objects is always presented, along with a standard set of representational objects. One possibility could be a teddy bear with blanket, bed, bottle, washcloth, and hairbrush, presented with blocks and objects of varying geometric shapes (e.g., cones, dowels, ovals, and circles), an assortment of balls, and a few sheets of paper. Either the SLP or the parent or guardian sits near the toys with the child and encourages him or her to complete a play theme (e.g., feeding the teddy bear and putting it to bed). The SLP ensures the use of both traditional, representational objects, such as the teddy bear and bed, and nonstandard objects in each play theme, occasionally encouraging substitution with the latter (e.g., giving the child a circle shape to represent a cookie, offering a sheet of paper in place of the blanket, etc.). The modeling of play, or imitative strategy, is an effective way of examining a child's zone of proximal development in the domain of play [27]. It has been repeatedly shown to elicit valid and reliable play behavior from typically developing children as well as children with a number of developmental delays [28-30]. However, the child should also be encouraged at some point in the evaluation to play alone with the set of objects so that one may compare his or her level and quality of play when alone, when with others, and when provided various forms of scaffolding. Furthermore, given that young children with developmental delays tend to demonstrate more variability in their play performances than do normally developing children, it is especially important to assess their play abilities based on repeated observations over time [31]. Each evaluation should be videotaped for later scoring.

It is essential to evaluate a child's play against the normal developmental sequence. In 1991, Casby [25] outlined the natural development of play using four developmental phases and described symbolic play in terms of its three major functional components: agent, instrument, and scheme [25] (See Table 1.) His model supports the premise that children of different developmental levels will play differently with the same toys. Performing a behavioral assessment with this model helps the SLP quantify emerging play skills as well as those that have been mastered.

Language Intervention Using Play as an Important Domain

Pretending and language are each, at their core, modes of symbolic thought. During pretend play, a block can stand in for a school bus. In language, letters and words represent concepts, objects, or events. Children practice creating symbols as they mentally transform objects during their play. Furthermore, the more time children spend pretending, the more opportunities they create to practice using language. During pretend play, children talk more, speak in lengthier utterances, and use more complex language (e.g., future tense, interrogative clauses, conditional verbs, descriptive adjectives, mental state verbs) than when engaged in other activities [32]. Moreover, Fisher [32] reported that a kindergartener's vocabulary correlates with the amount of time he or she spent talking with peers at three years of age during pretend play.

Table 1. Natural Development of Play

Phase	Age of Emergence	
Sensorimotor–Exploratory	2-4 months	Reaching, grasping, holding, rubbing, mouthing objects; repetitive pounding and hitting of objects
Relational–Nonfunctional	6-10 months	Relating objects to one another without regard for their social–conventional use (e.g., holding two or more objects, pushing objects together, stacking, bumping, nesting, offering objects to and taking objects from others)
Functional–Conventional	10-12 months	Relating objects to one another in a social–conventional manner; objects are used functionally in typical context (e.g., pushing toy car, scribbling with real crayon, putting cup on saucer, stirring bowl with spoon, feeding doll from toy bottle)
Symbolic – Agent – Self as the Agent	12-18 months	Child is both initiator and recipient of play actions (e.g., pretends to drink from a cup, pretends to talk on play telephone, brushes own hair during play cleaning/dressing)
Symbolic – Agent – Passive-Other	18-24 months	Child begins to use substitute agents but does not animate them (e.g., puts cup to doll's or teddy bear's mouth, puts telephone to teddy bear's mouth and ear, brushes doll's hair)

Table 1. (Continued)

Phase			Age of Emergence	
		Active-Other	24-30 months	Child animates substitute agents (e.g., makes drinking sounds while pretending doll or teddy bear is holding the cup to its mouth, speaks for teddy bear when it is "on the phone," pretends doll is brushing its own hair)
	Instrument	Realistic Object	10-12 months	Relating objects to one another in a social–conventional manner; objects are used functionally in typical context (e.g., pretending to drink from cup, pushing toy car, coloring with real crayon) *(See Functional-Conventional Phase.)*
		Substitute Object	18-24 months	Substituting another object for the standard one in play (e.g., using a cone as a rocket, pretending to use a block as a cup or a dowel as a crayon)
		Imaginary Object	24-30 months	Performing an object-action scheme without the use of an actual object (e.g., pretending to talk on an imaginary telephone, pretending to drink from an imaginary cup)
	Scheme	Single	12-18 months	Carrying out a single play act (e.g., guiding toy car, pretending to drink from cup and placing it on saucer)
		Multiple	18-24 months	Carrying out sequences of two or more play acts (e.g., pretending to cut food with knife, eat off plate with fork, and then drink from cup; pretending to comb own hair and then the hair of another)
		Complex/ Planned	about 30 months	Carrying out a sequence of theme-related play acts (e.g., cooking a pretend meal, setting a table for two, and then chatting with a doll over lunch)

In addition to language proficiency, pretend play contributes to a child's development of narrative abilities. The child must communicate his or her own ideas in joint creation of a play theme with their SLP. They also must integrate their SLP's ideas into a coherent narrative. Children may be better prepared to understand narratives when they have experienced or practiced similar concepts through play, such as creating descriptions to support a fantasy scenario. Through training in mature pretend play, children learn to use toys and props symbolically, develop narratives, maintain roles, and plan play scenarios from beginning to end [33].

Four key elements are needed to create the optimal early intervention treatment environment: (a) exposure, (b) deliberateness, (c) recurrence, and (d) responsiveness [31].

(a) Exposure refers to the linguistic input that is actively provided within the treatment setting. In some exposures, the child may be required to respond verbally and in others the child may be simply taking in the model of the appropriate linguistic structure. Children do not need to overtly produce or imitate language to acquire key language forms and concepts. Incidental exposures to language in a meaningful context can also be effective for language learning. (b) The SLPs are deliberate and intentional in the language that they choose. (c) Recurrence refers to the importance of repetition for children in acquiring linguistic concepts. For example, language delayed preschoolers require many opportunities to process new vocabulary. Through guided play, the highly skilled SLP provides many targeted learning experiences. (d) Responsiveness refers to the SLP's sensitivity to the child's developing communicative competencies. Responsiveness to children and use of child-initiated themes have repeatedly been associated with language gains in children [33].

Perhaps the most important aspect of intervention is to follow the child's lead. SLPs can observe what the child likes and dislikes and respond accordingly. They can also engage the child in theme-related conversations, ask questions, and respond to the child's ideas in a way that encourages use of targeted linguistic structures. A child may be struggling verbally during a conversation, but still be actively engaged and intrinsically motivated. At the mid-point between play and work, the child's motivation, coupled with guidance from the SLP, can create robust opportunities for language learning [34].

A language-rich treatment session involves SLPs who deliberately use language-stimulation strategies when interacting with children. Girolametto and Weitzman [34] identified eight key strategies that when used appropriately advance language development: waiting, pausing, confirming, imitating, extending, labeling, open questioning, and scripting.

- Waiting: Speak slowly and do not rush or dominate the conversation.
- Pausing: Encourage turn-taking during conversation and take care to be at eye-level with the child.
- Confirming: Respond to the child's interaction by commenting, smiling, and/or nodding.
- Imitating: Repeat what the child has stated in an affirming manner.
- Extending: Repeat the child's verbal responses and add verbal information. *Child*: I made a tower. *SLP*: You made a tall tower.
- Labeling: Label objects and object actions as well as feelings and reactions.
- Questions: Ask questions to encourage verbal interaction during play.
- Scripting: Describe the steps in a process. (e.g., "First you take the lid off the paint, then you carefully pour some in the tray, and then you can begin painting. Can you tell me what you do first?")

Table 2. Emerging Play with Corresponding Emerging Language

Emerging Play Level	Emerging Language Level
Child begins to involve relationships between objects as well as between objects and people. (Basis for object permanence; cause and effect)	*Content:* "first words" (e.g., more, in, out) *Form:* single words *Use:* joint attention
Child represents familiar activities of daily living by linking actions into a planned, multi-scheme sequence. Begins to substitute one object for another. *Example:* Child uses play block as bar of soap to wash puppy (stuffed animal), then wraps puppy in towel	*Content:* a variety of behavior-specific words (e.g., puppy, dirty, wash, dry) *Form:* single words as well as simple phrases and sentences, such as verb-object and subject-verb-object (e.g., "wash puppy", "I give bath.") *Use:* announcement of action

Girolametto, Weitzman [34] categorized these language stimulation techniques into child-oriented responses, interaction-promoting responses, and language-modeling responses. Justice [31] elaborated on the techniques: "Child–oriented responses, which are used to create and maintain a shared conversational focus between adult and child, include waiting and extending.

Interaction-promoting responses, which encourage the child into active dialogue, include pausing, open questioning, imitating, and confirming. Language–modeling responses provide children with demonstrations of linguistic forms, content and use. These responses include labeling and scripting." By using language stimulation techniques during play scenarios the SLP increases his or her responsiveness to the child's language competencies and provides the proper scaffolding to enhance language skills. In turn, the child learns to produce language that meets their individualized and targeted goals [34-39].

The steps of a language treatment session using play to extend language and new learning are listed below.

1. Arrange a setting that contains materials for play that are of interest to the child and are appropriate for the child's level of play.
2. Wait for the child to initiate an interaction about an object of interest.
3. Elaborate upon child responses.
4. Expand and extend the language and play, working on emerging objectives.

The Role of Parents and Caregivers

Parents and caregivers are often the child's first play partners. Starting in infancy, parents initiate play with children through simple games like peek-a-boo. By the child's second birthday, parents and children should regularly engage in pretend play. Early involvement from parents as initiators, directors, and partners in play serves to introduce children to more structured play by adding concepts and vocabulary that they would not be exposed to playing alone or with peers.

Guided play can take two forms. At a very basic level, parents can enrich their child's environment by providing objects or experiences that promote language learning. In the more direct form of guided play, parents can scaffold their child's play by joining in the fun as a co-player, asking thoughtful questions, commenting on children's discoveries, and encouraging further exploration. The idea that children can benefit from parent guidance and participation in play is empirically supported.

Table 3. Play Toolkit

Toy Complexity Continuum	
Cause and Effect	These toys are designed for a distinct effect (e.g., jack-in-the-box, ball-and-hammer toy)
Closed-Ended	Playing with these toys guides conversation along one avenue and involves a distinct beginning and end. (e.g., Mr./Mrs. Potato Head, ring stacker, puzzles)
Open-Ended	These toys never suggest completion and may lead conversation in any number of directions. (e.g., blocks, Legos, dollhouse)
Joint Play	These games are important for socialization. (e.g., follow-the-leader, duck duck goose, hide and seek, red light-green light)
Music/Song Games	(e.g., ring around the rosie, London bridges, parachute, the hokey pokey)
Turn-Taking Games	(e.g., bean bag toss, bowling games, board games)
Pretend Play	Child imagines his or herself into the play unfolding
	Performs sequences of actions within scenarios
	Role-plays with occupations, characters, animals, etc.
Play Centers/ Social Pretending	(e.g., doctor's office, grocery store, school, restaurant, camping)
Common Object Box	
Used for identifying, demonstrating, and naming objects and their functions	(e.g., farm animals, phone, keys, car, hat, shoe, sock, sunglasses, brush, ball, bowl, spoon, cup, book, etc.)
Pretend-Play Props	Boxes and containers of various shapes and sizes
	Dress-up clothes, shoes, hats, bags, and aprons
	Kitchen and household items, both toy and real (e.g., measuring cups, wooden spoons)
	Specialty items such as a doctor kit or a toy workbench and tools
	Puppets, stuffed animals, baby dolls, and caregiving items such as bottles, blankets, and diapers

In the clinical setting parents and caregivers are actively involved in observational learning, where they view and discuss treatment sessions with the SLP. If parents and primary caregivers are not able to attend treatment sessions, they can also learn language stimulation strategies by viewing their child's video-taped treatment sessions.

CONCLUSION

In summary, play is an important domain for the assessment and treatment of delayed language development in infants and children. However, there is a long standing tradition in play research of focusing primarily on free play. The majority of studies have been done in naturalistic settings with children engaged in free play and little or no adult responsiveness or clinical intervention. The limited research concerning early play, cognitive and language development has consistently found compelling correlations. Further research is needed to examine the benefits to language delayed children of early, developmentally appropriate, intensive language therapy in a play-based environment.

REFERENCES

[1] Neeley, P.M., Neeley, R.A., Justen, J.E. III, Tipton-Sumner, C. (2001). Scripted play as a language intervention strategy for preschoolers with developmental disabilities. *Early Childhood Education Journal* 28, (4).

[2] Odom, S.L., McConnell, S.R., Brown, W.H. (2008). Social competence of children: Conceptualizations, assessment, and influences. Baltimore, MD: Brookes, 3-30.

[3] Casby, M.W. (1997). Symbolic play of children with language impairment: a critical review. *Journal of Speech, Language, and Hearing Research* 40, 468-479.

[4] Guralnick, M.J. (1999). The nature and. meaning of social integration of young children with mild developmental delays in inclusive settings. *Journal of Early Intervention* 22,70-86.

[5] Roskos, K., Christie, J. (2011). The play-literacy nexus and the importance of evidence-based techniques in the classroom. *American Journal of Play* (2): 204-224.

[6] Leong, D.J., Bodrova, E. (2014). Why children need play. *Scholastic Early Childhood Today.*

[7] Piaget, J., Inhelder, B. (1969). The psychology of the child. General Publishing Co.

[8] Bates, E. (1989). Integrating language and gesture in infancy. *Developmental Psychology,* 25, (6),1004-1019.

[9] Lifter, K., Bloom, L. (1989). Object play and the emergence of language. *Infant Behavior and Development.* 12, (4), 395-423.

[10] McCune, L., Nicholich, L. (1981). Toward symbolic functioning: Structure of early pretend games and potential parallels with language. *Child Development.* 52, 785-797.

[11] McCune, L. (1995). A normative study of representational play at the transition to language. *Developmental Psychology.* 31, 198-206.

[12] Piaget, J. (1959). The language and thought of the child. *Psychology Press.*

[13] Rossetti, L. (2001). Communication intervention: Birth to three (2nd ed.). San Diego, California: *Singular.*

[14] Casby, M.W. (2003). The development of symbolic play in children. *Communication Disorders Quarterly,* 24, 175-183.

[15] Lifter, K., Bloom, L. (1998). *Intentionality and the role of play in the transition to language.* In Wetherby, A.M., Warren, S.F., Reichle, J. (Eds.), *Transitions in prelinguistic communication: Preintentional to intentional and presymbolic to symbolic,* Brookes, 161-198.

[16] Bates, E. Benigni, L., Bretherton, I., Camaioni, L., Volterra, V. (1979). *The emergence of symbols: Cognition and communication in infancy.* New York: Academic Press.

[17] Bates, E., Bretherton, I., Snyder, L., Shore, C., Volterra, V. (1980). *Vocal and gestural symbols at 13 months.* Merrill-Palmer Quarterly, 26, 407-423.

[18] Casby, M.W., Della Corte, M. (1987). *Symbolic play performance and early language development.* Journal of Psycholinguistic Research, 16, 312-42.

[19] Roth, F.P., Clark, D.M., (1987). *Symbolic play and social participation abilities of language-impaired and normally developing children.* Journal of Speech and Hearing Disorders, 52(1): 17-29.

[20] Terrell, B.Y., Schwartz, R.G. (1988). *Object transformation in the play of language impaired children.* Journal of Speech and Hearing Disorders, 53, 449-456.

[20] Robbins, D.L., Fein, D., Barton, M., Green, J.A. (2009). *The modified checklist for autism in toddlers (M-CHAT-R/F).* American Academy of Pediatrics.

[21] Fenson et al. (2007). *The Mcarthur-Bates communicative development inventories.* Brookes Publishing Co.

[22] Sigman, M., McGovern, C.W., (2005). *Improvement in cognitive and language skills from preschool to adolescence in autism.* Journal of Autism and Developmental Disorders, 35(1) 15-23.

[23] Bopp, K.D., Smith,V., Mirenda, P. (2006). *Predictors of development in autism.* www.asha.org. [22006.

[24] Casby, M.W., Ruder, K.F. (1983). *Symbolic play and early language development in normal and mentally retarded children.* Journal of Speech and Hearing Research. 26(3): 404-411.

[25] Casby, M.W. (1991a). *Symbolic play: A developmental framework.* Infant-Toddler Intervention, 1, 219-231.

[26] Casby, M.W. (1991 b). *Symbolic play: A unified model.* Infant-Toddler Intervention, 1, 233-243.

[27] Vygotsky, L. (1978). *Mind in society: The development of higher psychological processes.*

[28] Fenson, L., Ramsey, D. (1980). *Decentration and integration of the child's play in the second year.* Child Development, 51, 171-178.

[29] Riguet, C., Taylor, N., Benaroya, S., Klein, L. (1981). *Symbolic play in autistic, Down Syndrome, and normal children of equivalent mental age.* Journal of Autism and Developmental Disorders, 11, 439-448.

[30] Watson, M., Fischer, K. (1980). *Development of social roles in elicited and spontaneous behavior during the preschool years.* Developmental Psychology, 16, 483-494.

[31] Justice, L. M., (2002). *A team-based action plan for creating language-rich preschool classroom environments.* University of Virginia/justice.teambasedaction.pdf.

[32] Fisher, K., Hirsch-Pasek, K., Golinkoff, R. M., Singer, D. G. (2011). *Playing around in school: Implications for learning and educational policy.* In A. Pellegrini (Ed.), The Oxford handbook of the development of play (pp. 341-362). New York: Oxford University Press.

[33] White, R.E., (2012). *The power of play.* Minnesota Children's Museum. www.mcm.org

[34] Girolametto, L., Weitzman, E. (2002). *Responsiveness of child care providers in interactions with toddlers and preschoolers.* lshss.pubs.asha.org/article.aspx?articleid=1780291.

[35] Gronlund, G. (2010). *Developmentally appropriate play: Guiding young children to a higher level.* St Paul, MN: Redleaf Press

[36] Tools of the Mind (2012). Tools of the Mind website. http://www. toolsofthemind.org

[37] Bodrova, E., Leong, D., Atwill, K., Ko, L., & Saifer, S. (2009, April). *Scaffolding intentional make-believe play and the development of self-regulation: Results from the Tools of the Mind program*. Society for the Research of Child Development. Denver, Colorado.

[38] Chapman, R. S., (2000). *Children's language learning: An interactionist perspective.* Journal of Child Psychology and Psychiatry, 41, 33-54.

[39] Bloom, L., Tinker, E., (2001). *The intentionality model and language acquisition.* Monographs of the Society for Research in Child Development, 66.

In: Speech, Language and Voice Pathology ISBN: 978-1-63321-958-8
Editor: Pablo Antonio Ysunza

Chapter 5

THE IMPACT OF PROTRACTED PHONOLOGICAL DISORDERS ON LITERACY OUTCOMES IN CHILDREN: A META-ANALYSIS

Glenda Kelly Mason* and Barbara May Bernhardt
The University of British Columbia. Vancouver, Canada

ABSTRACT

Background: The literature is equivocal on whether children with protracted phonological development (PPD) are at risk for literacy acquisition, making it challenging to provide relevant evidence-based phonological intervention. Differences in researchers' definitions of PPD have possibly contributed to the contradictory outcomes.

Purpose: The purpose of the meta-analysis was to determine the consistency of word-level literacy differences for children with and without PPD, and whether such differences are moderated by definitions of PPD.

Method: Eligible studies had measured at least one word-level literacy construct in school-aged children with and without PPD. Fifty-two evaluated papers generated 64 independent samples to examine: *Phonological awareness* (*PA*; n = 20), *Word decoding* (*DEC*; n = 17), *Fluency* (*FL*; n = 4), *Nonword decoding* (*NWD*; n = 9) and *Spelling* (*SP*;

* Email: g.kellmas@alumni.ubc.ca.

n = 14). Multiple regression analysis of a model that included all constructs was significant, $F(4,60) = 85.96$, $p < .001$ ($t = 5.71$, $p < .001$). Sample sizes allowed moderator testing for *PA*, *DEC*, *NWD*, and *SP*. A random effects model was used to compare *mean unbiased d* (weighted by the *inverse variance* and *Random Effects Variance Component*) on the *Q*-statistic ($p < .05$).

Results: For *unbiased Cohen's d, 95% Confidence Intervals* and *95% Credibility Intervals* were significant for *PA* ($d = .85$), *NWD* ($d = .50$), and *SP* ($d = .84$), but not *DEC* ($d = .63$) and *FL* ($d = 3.04$). Cultural context was a significant moderator of *SP*, suggesting dialectical influences. In defining PPD, age at literacy evaluation, severity/sub-type and resolution of PPD significantly moderated *NWD* ($Q = 14.21$) and *SP* ($Q = 8.00$). Complexity of speech context, particularly inclusion of multisyllabic word (MSW) evaluations, was a significant moderator of *PA* ($Q = 4.85$), *DEC* ($Q = 4.14$) and *SP* ($Q = 5.66$). Differences between children with and without PPD were greater in initial phases of childhood literacy compared with later phases.

Conclusions: In both initial and later phases of childhood literacy, early spoken phonological intervention seemed relevant to mitigating differences between children with and without PPD, although results were limited by the number of studies examined. To define PPD, spoken MSW phonology appeared important; a theoretically grounded continuous metric could increase study power, whether or not categorical samples are available.

Keywords: Literacy; Multisyllabic words; Phonology; Phonological awareness; Phonological disorders; Protracted phonological development; Reading; Speech delay; Speech sound disorders; Spelling; Typical phonological development

INTRODUCTION

Over the past two decades, a number of studies have evaluated the relationship between phonological development and literacy outcomes. [1-14] Research evidence concerning the relationship between phonological and literacy development provides a foundation for clinicians providing therapy to children with difficulties in either or both areas. A meta-analysis was conducted for the current chapter on this topic, examining studies that included children with typical versus protracted phonological development. The term *Protracted Phonological Development* (*PPD*) encompasses various other terms in the literature, including: (a) combinations of *Phonological, Speech*

Sound, (In)Consistent Speech, (Developmental) Speech, or Articulation, with one of *Disorder, Impairment, Delay, or Errors*; and (b) *Developmental Verbal Apraxia* or *Childhood Apraxia of Speech*. For the various studies, researchers typically sampled SLP caseloads of children with clinical diagnoses of protracted phonological development (PPD), the majority having received phonological intervention. However, an examination of the studies shows contradictory literacy outcomes that at least in part seemed to reflect differences in research methodology. These methodological differences include broader developmental considerations such as age at literacy evaluation and co-occurrence of other conditions, such as *Protracted Language Development (PLD).*

In particular, children designated with severe or persistent PPD appeared to have lower literacy outcomes than those with less severe PPD. [15-17] Thus, differences in participant selection, possibly reflecting researchers' definitions of PPD, might subsequently have contributed to the apparent contradictions.

Thus, for the meta-analysis discussed in the current chapter, a variety of methodological parameters were examined relative to age of literacy acquisition and characterization of PPD through traditional severity rankings, sub-types, resolution, and the complexity of speech context assessed. While accounting for association with PLD, therapy history and other differences in study design, the analysis aimed to (a) summarize and quantify literacy outcomes, and (b) statistically explain the variation in these outcomes in terms of age and the selected PPD parameters.

In addition to selecting participant variables related to age and characterization of PPD, relevant literacy outcomes were identified. Spoken phonology is reported to be directly related to word level literacy but only indirectly to comprehension. [18, 19]

Thus, the meta-analysis examined literacy constructs most likely connected to the cognitive organization of the speech sound system: (a) phonological awareness, (b) word decoding, (c) fluency, (d) nonword decoding, and (e) spelling. As background, the following sections describe key parameters for the analysis: characterization and evaluation of PPD and literacy constructs included, and literacy outcomes for children with protracted versus typical phonological development.

LITERACY AND THE CHARACTERIZATION OF PROTRACTED PHONOLOGICAL DEVELOPMENT

Authors have noted an overlap of PPD, Protracted Language Development (PLD), and lags in literacy attainment, [2, 20, 21] which Peterson, McGrath, Smith and Pennington (2007) [22] suggest could arise from a shared risk factor for phonological deficits, but also factors unique to each. Studies of children with PPD, in the absence of co-occurring PLD, have demonstrated inconsistency relative to literacy outcomes, with some results showing low risk, [6, 23, 24] and others, high risk. [8, 25] Researchers have reported the lowest literacy outcomes for children described as having more severe or persistent PPD. [16, 26] However, the characterization of PPD and its relative severity differ across the studies.

These differing perspectives on PPD have concerned the relevance of: (a) continuous [27] versus discrete categories of severity [28] versus sub-types of PPD [29, 30, 31]; (b) resolution or persistence of PPD [10, 32]; and (c) evaluation method with respect to both elicitation type (single-word versus connected speech), [33] and word complexity (primarily mono- and di-syllabic words versus multisyllabic). [34] Word complexity might also be relevant for characterization of PPD as *resolved*; if insufficient numbers of MSWs were tested, ongoing difficulty with timing and sequencing of both syllables and speech sounds may have been missed, at least up to the age of 7 years. [35]

Further to word complexity, production of MSWs may be a key component in evaluation of the relationships between spoken phonology and literacy. Researchers have shown relationships between MSW production, phonological awareness skills, fluent word or nonword decoding, and spelling. For example, Core (2004) [37] identified positive correlations between phonological awareness scores and Percent Consonants Correct (PCC) on a MSW naming task in 5- and 6-year-olds. Larrivee and Catts (1999) [26] observed that MSW and nonword repetition in children with severe PPD at the end of kindergarten, predicted outcomes in decoding and nonword decoding at the end of grade 1, and explained the greatest variance in decoding (including MSW *DEC*) in grade 3. [38] For ages 5 to 8;7 years, PCC of MSWs explained a larger significant unique variance in composite real and nonword decoding when included in a model with composite phonological awareness and lexical retrieval scores. [39]

In addition to such differences in characterization of PPD, diversity in terms of literacy construct and/or measurement method are relevant in evaluation of the relationship between PPD and literacy.

CHARACTERIZATION OF LITERACY AND THE INCLUDED CONSTRUCTS

In terms of literacy evaluation, the stage of acquisition is relevant. In earlier elementary school, formal literacy instruction begins and focuses chiefly on the letter names, sound-symbol correspondence and basic spelling patterns needed to decode frequent words. In later elementary school, literacy instruction places a greater emphasis on extracting meaning from text, which comprises words with decreasing frequency. In the high school years and beyond, students must decode and comprehend infrequent multimorphemic words, and comprehend increasingly abstract text in the context of less explicit literacy instruction. [40] Theories of literacy strive to account for student advancement across these stages, with word level literacy considered a foundation for all of them. [41]

Most theories assume spoken and print language to be connected through some aspect of phonological processing, particularly the representation of smaller speech units by letters. [42, 43] The commonly described *Dual Route* models suggest that reading or spelling words involves two separate cognitive procedures. [44, 45] The models aim to explain how knowledge of word sub-units (phonological awareness) enables reading of familiar versus unfamiliar words (word and nonword decoding) and their orthographic encoding (spelling). However, the constructs and evaluation of phonological awareness, decoding and spelling have also varied across studies, discussed as follows.

Phonological Awareness (PA)

Phonological awareness (PA) refers to knowledge (implicit and explicit) that words are composed of sub-units (e.g., syllable, onset, rhyme, phoneme), and to the ability to consciously manipulate these units mentally. [4, 46, 47] Studies have shown robust relationships between word level literacy and *PA*, [18, 48, 49] with a minimum proficiency deemed necessary for acquiring phonological to orthographic correspondences for both monosyllabic, [50] and MSW word recognition. [51]

Characterization and evaluation of *PA* have differed in conjunction with children's developmental level. Task characterization has varied in terms of levels of meta-cognitive awareness and working memory, language recognition versus production, and the size of phonological units. [13, 46, 52, 53] Studies have utilized standardized tests, [1, 39, 47] nonstandardized tasks, [12, 36, 53] or a combination thereof. [8, 11] Rhyme and onset matching tasks have predominated through age 6 years. For 7- to 8-year-olds, segmenting and blending have been common, sometimes of syllables and onsets but more often, phonemes. Phoneme manipulation tasks have frequently been administered from age 7 years, initially elision, and progressing to phoneme reversals at ages 10 through 13 years.

Decoding (DEC) and Fluency (FL)

In terms of word reading, Ehri (1992) [49] described the relationship between dual routes for recognizing words, i.e., *recoding* or *decoding (DEC),* and automatic sight recognition, *fluency (FL). DEC* is assumed to rely on intermediate application of grapheme-to-phoneme rules for translation of orthographic representations into suprasegmental structure and phonological segments, before accessing meaning. [41] As reading proficiency increases, readers learn progressively larger orthographic chunks, including syllabic patterns, with few exposures to a word. This enhances *FL*, suggesting stronger and faster cognitive connections from orthography to phonology and meaning. [49] All orthographic words may in fact connect to meaning and pronunciation concurrently, [44, 54, 55] emphasizing the foundation of accurate spoken phonology for translating print into speech. [56, 57]

Nonword Decoding (NWD)

In *nonword decoding* (*NWD*), knowledge of grapheme-to-phoneme rules is required to read pseudowords, and so is largely accomplished without the contribution of meaning. [54] As children develop representations of larger chunks of orthographic patterns, however, word neighborhoods might aid in recognition of parts of nonwords. [41] In child literacy development, the importance of *NWD* has come from evidence that acquisition of phoneme-to-grapheme correspondences depends on factors beyond phonological awareness (e.g., some children have performed well on *PA* tasks but not on tasks involving phonological to orthographic correspondence). [50]

In comparison with the variety of *PA* assessments, *DEC* and *NWD* have been primarily assessed on word lists from standardized tests, [53, 58] and infrequently on nonstandardized tasks. [2, 58] Standardized tests of *DEC* have been created in several contexts: North America, [8, 14] Great Britain, [2, 31] Australia, [4] and New Zealand. [5] Uniquely, Overby et al. (2012) [7] determined the ecological validity of measures from the Templin Archive (2004) of longitudinal data from 1960-1972. Irrespective of country, the *Word Attack* subtest of the *Woodcock Reading Mastery Test* [59, 60] was the standardized measure used to evaluate *NWD*. [1, 5, 14, 24] The few studies investigating *FL* varied as to whether primary or secondary data were collected, from a small sample of word and nonword list evaluations [12] to a large database of passage reading assessments, [10] respectively.

Spelling (SP)

Turning to the final construct, *spelling (SP)* requires representation of spoken words with conventional orthography. [61] Neuroimaging studies about accuracy and reaction time for regular, irregular and nonword *SP* recognition have supported both phonological and lexical routes for spelling. [62] Because accurate, as opposed to phonologically legal spelling, must be generated, [45, 63] *SP* possibly relies on more detailed, explicit phonological to orthographic connections than reading. Ehri (1992) [49] considered such full alphabetic skill to be hierarchically organized, with automaticity gained from strong long-term memory connections between *SP* and pronunciation. Representing words in print is further taxed by demands for coordination with fine motor output, integration with morphosyntactics and, if in text versus list form, organization of ideas.

In studies of children with PPD, *SP* has been uniformly assessed using word dictation but with various measures, including recently standardized tests, [6, 36, 64] older standardized tests, [2, 4, 7, 65] and nonstandardized tasks. [1, 5, 32]

Literacy Outcomes

Keeping in mind the diversity in characterization and evaluation of PPD and literacy, the following section provides an overview of literacy comparisons between children with and without PPD as background for the meta-analysis. The term PPD will pertain to any diagnosed history, whether or not considered ongoing at the point of literacy measurement. Thus, the groups studied will be stratified only by age to highlight progression with literacy.

Phonological Awareness (PA)

Studies of *PA* have compared children with typical versus protracted phonological development in the early and late elementary school years, i.e., *learning to read* and *reading to learn* phases, respectively. [40] Preschoolers with PPD (3- to 6-year-olds), have shown lags on composite score analyses, [11, 37, 46] and awareness or matching subtests at the rhyme and word initial phoneme levels, [4, 12, 53] with significance on whole word segmentation and blending. [52, 47] In late preschool, at 5 to 6 years of age, persistent PPD has had the strongest relationship with *PA* and a moderate *effect size* (*ES*). [11]

At school age, studies have focused on the *learning to read* phase. Six- to eight-year-olds with PPD history have shown equivalence to children with TD on rhyme and phoneme awareness but significantly lower scores on various phoneme segmentation and blending tasks. [13, 58, 66] On the latter tasks, children up to age 9 years have scored within the average range, yet shown significant differences compared with TD children. [1] Peterson et al. (2009) [8] also found a significant difference and large *ES* on a *PA* composite for 7- to 9-year-olds; furthermore, controlling for nonverbal IQ, persistent PPD at age four years predicted ongoing *PA* difficulty.

Fewer studies have compared *PA* outcomes for older school-aged children or adolescents with PPD history versus typical development. Also uncommon are studies evaluating longer words or manipulation tasks, such as elision or substitution of segments. School-aged children with and without PPD, predominantly 8- to 11-year-olds, have performed equally well on blending and segmentation tasks but with ceiling effects. [6, 36, 38] On more advanced *PA* tasks of manipulation, such as reversed phoneme segmentation or Pig Latin, adolescents with PPD have lagged behind TD peers, irrespective of significance levels. [2, 9] However, the relationship of such tasks to literacy is unclear.

Overall, children with PPD history from preschool through adolescence appear to lag behind TD children on *PA* composites or subtests of increasing complexity. *Effect sizes* suggest moderate to large differences. Finally, PPD in early childhood is associated with lower *PA* outcomes, which in turn have predicted ongoing *PA* difficulty.

Decoding Skills: *Word Decoding (DEC), Nonword Decoding (NWD)* and *Fluency (FL)*

Outcomes for decoding skills have been reported for the *learning to read* phase, and to a lesser extent, the *reading to learn* phase. In each phase, whether or not significant, lower scores have been reported for children with PPD than for those without. In the initial phase, despite ceiling effects, 5- to 7; 6-year-olds with PPD have shown significantly lower scores on *DEC* and *NWD* than TD peers. [2, 58, 67] Other studies have found average, but lower scores for children with PPD compared with those of their TD peers, with both significant, [7] and non-significant differences. [4, 23, 24]

Within wider age ranges, 6- to 9-year-olds with PPD have also had average achievement on *DEC*, [1, 8] and in comparison with children with TD, superior performance has been reported for *NWD* subsequent to PA therapy, with a large *ES*. [5] More broadly, small samples of school children aged 7 to 11 years showed significantly lower *DEC* scores, [31, 65] but using an upper limit of 13 years, *DEC* and *NWD* have been within average. [14, 68] Adolescents aged 12 to 17 years have also obtained average but consistently lower scores on *DEC* and *NWD*. [36]

A final aspect of decoding is *fluency*. For children with PPD, few studies of this construct exist, and those that do have focused mainly on the *learning to read* phase. For 5- to 6-year-olds with PPD, performance on words and nonwords has been in the average range, but significantly lower for the nonwords. [12] Meredith (2002) [6] found average word *FL* for 8- to 9-year-olds with PPD but with significant differences and large *ESs* compared with children with TD. [6] Finally, by grades 2 to 3, *FL* in connected text has been negatively correlated with persisting PPD. [8, 10]

To summarize the findings for the decoding attainment of school-age children with PPD history, average performance has been demonstrated on *DEC*, *NWD* and *FL,* although this performance may lag behind that of groups with TD. As was implied for *PA, ESs* suggest moderate to large magnitudes of difference for decoding, nonword repetition and fluency.

Spelling (SP)

More consistent results have been reported regarding *SP* proficiency, where children with history of PPD have performed significantly lower than their TD counterparts, [2, 7, 32] even during adolescence. [36, 68] A history of PPD has also predicted unique significant variance in *SP*. [1] Nonetheless, some studies have shown performance within the average range for children with history of PPD. [6, 7, 68]

MOTIVATION AND QUESTIONS FOR THE META-ANALYSIS

Assuming equivalence between children with and without PPD in other developmental domains, the overall disadvantages in word level literacy of children with PPD are important for at least two reasons: (a) decoding of longer infrequent words and comprehension of increasingly abstract text might become more challenging, and consequently, (b) the range of available educational, career or employment choices might be narrower than for TD children.

The synopsis above suggests that overall, children with PPD history have lower literacy outcomes than their TD peers, even when their scores fall within the average range of tests normed on typically developing children. However, questions remain concerning the scale of difference for the selected word level constructs, the relative contributions of earlier versus later phases of childhood acquisition (*learning to read* versus *reading to learn*), and characterization and evaluation of PPD. A meta-analysis was thus undertaken in order to address those topics in terms of the following questions:

1. Are children with PPD consistently disadvantaged in word level literacy acquisition compared with TD peers, and if so, to what extent? Moderate to large magnitudes of difference were predicted between children with and without PPD, for each literacy construct: *Phonological Awareness, Decoding, Nonword Decoding* and *Spelling,* with the greatest group differences in *Spelling*.
2. Are there between-group differences in both the early (*learning to read*) and later (*reading to learn*) childhood phases of literacy acquisition? Between-group differences were predicted in both phases.

3. Are there differences between school-aged children with and without PPD that vary according to the characterization of PPD? The degree of protracted phonological development at time of literacy measurement was predicted to explain differences between groups whether envisioned as discrete categories of severity and sub-type, or resolution of PPD. Variation in methods used to characterize PPD, in terms of context of assessment, (i.e., MSWs and connected speech) was predicted to explain between-group differences.

METHOD

This section first briefly describes the meta-analytic objectives, and then outlines steps for the current analysis, including: search methods and study inclusion criteria, coding of moderators and reliability, data selection and transformation for *effect size* (*ES*) calculations, and methods for obtaining descriptive and analytic results.

Meta-analysis Objectives

Meta-analysis provides a statistical synthesis of comprehensive research findings obtained from different study designs and/or from sub-sets of data within studies. [69, 70, 71] The included studies/data serve as the participants upon which hypotheses are tested. *Effect sizes* (the magnitude and direction of actual differences) calculated from the selected data are standardized in order to aggregate and compare them. The method involves transformations, weighting and fitting of data to a statistical equation that takes into account study influence by sample size. These processes address bias arising from the sampling of studies, and/or the populations from which samples within studies are taken. While primary investigations explain variability in results according to dependent variables, meta-analyses examine independent variables (moderators) of interest and potentially specify gaps in research.

Study Selection

To obtain a comprehensive sample of studies of literacy outcomes for children with PPD, search terms included school age/ children/ childhood/

SSD/ speech/ articulation/ phonological/ disorders/ disabilities/ impairment / apraxia of speech/ phonological awareness/ literacy/ decoding/ word decoding/ word recognition/ fluency/ nonword decoding/ spelling/ comprehension/ reading/ dyslexia. The search for peer reviewed primary articles, conference proceedings and dissertations for any year included the main speech-language pathology, applied linguistics and education databases: Academic Search Complete, Cochrane Systematic Reviews, Communication and Mass Media Complete, CINAHL (Cumulative Index to Nursing and Allied Health Literature), Dissertation Abstracts International, Education Full Text (H.W. Wilson), Education Index Retrospective: 1929-1983 (H.W. Wilson), Education Research Complete, ERIC (Education Resource Information Center), Linguistics and Language Behavior Abstracts (LLBA), PsycARTICLES, PsycBOOKS, PsycINFO, PsycEXTRA, and Pub Med (1946-present). Subsequently, 5128 abstracts were reviewed (including duplicates in the various databases), from which 52 papers were evaluated, and their reference lists searched for additional candidates.

Inclusion Criteria

Inclusion criteria were relevant to aspects of study design, participant socio-behavioral characteristics, and available *effect size (ES)* data. Included studies measured at least one literacy construct of interest, in school-aged monolingual English-speaking children with PPD history (without other notable developmental conditions) and a typically developing comparison group (TD).

With respect to data availability, *ESs* (or means and standard deviations from which to calculate *ESs*) either had to be published or obtainable from authors. Thirty-four studies, reported from 1980 to 2012, met the inclusion criteria, generating 64 independent samples distributed across constructs accordingly: *PA* n = 20; *DEC* n = 17; *FL* n = 4; *NWD* n = 9; and *SP* n = 14. A total of 4007 children from 4 to 17 years old (1496 with PPD and 2511 with TD) was represented, with construct and corresponding sample sizes as follows: *PA* n = 994 (n_{PPD} = 527, n_{TD} = 467); *DEC* n = 1717 (n_{PPD} = 410, n_{TD} = 1307); *FL* n = 10455 (n_{PPD} = 1520, n_{TD} = 8935); *NWD* n = 479 (n_{PPD} = 206, n_{TD} = 273); and *SP* n = 817 (n_{PPD} = 353, n_{TD} = 464). Few age spans were as narrow as one year: an age span of 3 to 3½ years and 4½ to 5½ years was reported by 50% and 40% of studies, respectively; in one study, the range was 6½ years.

In some cases, data clarifications and adjustments were needed before *ESs* could be determined. Clarifications included: (a) establishing sample independence in Holm et al., 2008 [4] (A. Holm, personal communication, November 22, 2011); (b) verifying a reading correlation value in Overby et al., 2012 [7] (M. Overby, personal communication, February 27, 2012); and (c) obtaining unpublished data for Apel & Lawrence (2011) [1], Sutherland & Gillon (2006) [47], and Wellman et al. (2011) [14]. Catts (1991) and (1993) [23, 24] were treated as one longitudinal study because the second study followed up on the sample of children in the first. Finally, to improve equivalence of data and reduce the number of inferential tests for *PA,* composite scores were calculated if unreported, e.g., Peterson et al., 2009. [8]

Coding of Included Studies

Coding was pertinent to the inclusion criteria and also to: publication identity, participant socio-behavioral attributes, literacy measures, and PPD characterization with consideration of co-occurring PLD. Coded socio-behavioral attributes were those used by researchers to equate comparison groups (and in some cases, tested for equivalence post hoc). [2, 11] Attributes considered were age, and one or more of the following: grade, classroom, IQ, language skills, reading/spelling level (when not a dependent literacy variable), ethnicity and SES/maternal education. Specific tests of each literacy construct were also coded.

In relation to characterization of PPD, exclusion of additional studies on the basis of potential bias arising from co-occurring PLD was also judged. The proportion of co-occurring PLD within included samples was coded for and language evaluation methods were reviewed. Whereas a small percentage of studies referred to a clinical history without PLD diagnosis, 85% directly assessed language performance across a variety of comprehension and/or production skills. In the latter case, co-occurring PLD was defined by accepted clinical criteria (1.5 SD below the mean or criterion cut-off) and/or a significant post hoc comparison between groups with and without PPD. Analysis of these methods for identifying co-occurring PLD suggested that a third of included studies (40% of those studies that directly evaluated PLD) reported no more than 25% co-occurring PLD. The coders agreed, therefore, that there was reasonable control for confounding of literacy outcomes by co-occurring PLD, and no further studies were excluded.

Following examination of co-occurring PLD, PPD was characterized in terms of status and evaluation parameters. Statuses at time of diagnosis and at literacy measurement were coded with respect to: (a) traditional severity ratings, (b) subtype frameworks such as pattern consistency or *Childhood Apraxia of Speech* (*CAS*), and (c) resolution or persistence. With respect to resolution, mixed groups were coded as persistent if investigators reported few children with resolved PPD (e.g., 3 of 15 in Catts, 1993 [24]; 7 of 86 in Peterson et al., 2009 [8]). Coded evaluation parameters were the specific testing methods used, elicitation type (single words, connected speech) and word complexity (mono- and disyllabic versus multisyllabic). Coding of word complexity took into account that: (a) prominent stress occurs more commonly on word-initial syllables in English disyllabic (DSW) words; (b) adult-like production of DSWs with weak (unstressed) initial syllables presents a notable challenge in childhood phonological acquisition; [27] and (c) DSWs with initial unstressed syllables and MSWs, defined as three or more syllables, are infrequent on common norm-referenced tests (occurring less than 10% of the time). [35] Consequently, a dedicated corpus of MSWs was coded whenever researchers evaluated an independent set of at least ten DSWs with initial unstressed syllables and/or MSWs (the minimum number used in the included studies). [29, 72] Tests with fewer than 10% complex words, e.g., the often-used *Goldman Fristoe Test of Articulation* (*GFTA*), [73] were coded for mono- and di-syllabic words; otherwise, a mixture of mono-, di- and multi-syllabic words was coded. MSWs were not coded for connected speech elicitation, because type/token frequencies were unreported.

Reliability of Coding

Two Canadian certified and registered speech-language pathologists coded study moderators and *ES* data: (a) the first author, a doctoral student with dedicated coursework in meta-analysis and over 30 years of clinical experience, and (b) an SLP, holding a Master's degree with completed research project relating to PPD, and four years of clinical experience. Coding definitions were discussed, and when not agreed upon, the first author's coding stood. The correlation and degree of agreement for multiple coders rating multiple moderators was estimated with the *intraclass correlation (ICC)*. [74] Because both coders coded all moderators, and to allow greater generalizability to other pairs of coders, the *ICC* was tested in a fully crossed random effects design. High reliability on all study moderators was indicated,

ICC(2,1) = .976 [CI = .974-.978]. Regarding data selection and *ES* calculation reliability, differences were discussed to achieve 100% agreement.

Determination and Analysis of *ESs*

This section outlines the methods for the next three stages of the meta-analysis, beginning with obtaining *ESs* for the selected data, followed by the descriptive and then inferential analyses. The descriptive analysis applies to the distribution and weighting of *ESs*. The inferential process includes multiple regression analyses (MRAs) for identifying significant variability in any literacy construct, and subsequent testing of that variance on the selected moderators.

Calculation of *Cohen's d*

To allow examination of the standardized magnitudes (thus independent of sample size) of actual mean differences between groups with and without PPD, *Cohen's d* was the selected *ES* for the meta-analysis. To insure independence of samples, one *ES* per literacy construct per study was chosen. For calculation of *d,* weighted means and/or pooled standard errors (i.e., proportionate to comparison group sizes) were derived from available raw scores, gains, percentiles, and standard scores. Because the value of *d* tends to be upwardly biased in small samples, by applying conversion formulas, [75] accuracy was adjusted to *unbiased d,* which was used in all subsequent analyses.

Descriptive Analysis

In the first step of the descriptive analysis, distributions of *unbiased d* were assessed through construction of funnel plots, which allow for the greater variance in small samples, reducing the number of outliers. The second step was to adjust *unbiased d* to obtain more precise estimates of the population *ESs,* and adjust study influence relative to sample size. To obtain this *weighted d*, *unbiased d* was weighted by the inverse variance. [75] The adjustment contributed to retention of outliers, and thus, all of the data in the inferential analyses. The magnitude of *weighted d* was interpreted according to Cohen's

(1988) [76] conventions (small ≥ 2; medium ≥ 5; large ≥ 8). For the *z-test* of the significance of each study *ES* and the mean for each construct, *95% Confidence Intervals* (*CI*) were constructed.

Inferential Analysis

Moving to the inferential analysis, two MRAs (p <.05) were conducted to determine if any of the constructs had significant variance to explain by the testing of moderators. In the first regression, a fixed effects model (which assumes that all possible studies are included) analyzed *weighted ds*. However, the analyzed studies were likely estimating for different populations because of: (a) a small sample of *ESs* per construct; (b) limitations in attaining sample size power through random sampling of children with PPD; and (c) variation in parameters used to equate comparison groups. The MRA was therefore repeated on the *mixed weighted ESs* using a random effects model (which assumes that all possible studies are not included). This entailed re-weighting of the *weighted ds* by adding the *Random Effects Variance Component* (*REVC*), i.e., the variability across possible populations of study samples. The additional weighting yielded a more stringent regression because the resultant *95% Credibility Interval (CredInt)* for the *mixed weighted d* could be expected to increase (more likely to contain zero), potentially decreasing the number of significant *ESs*.

Testing of Moderators

In this last stage of the meta-analysis, for each significant literacy construct, two groups of *mixed weighted ESs* were compared on a selected moderator by a *Q*-ANOVA (based on *Chi-square* for categorical variables, similar to 1-way ANOVA), $p < .05$. The result indicated whether the grouping variable (moderator) accounted for significant variability and whether there was significant variability (heterogeneity) remaining to be explained by other moderators. This process of testing moderators continued until either: (a) homogeneity of variances (no additional significant variance) was reached; (b) all moderators of interest had been tested; or (c) there were insufficient *ESs* (for the current meta-analysis, n < 3) to allow further meaningful analysis.

To address more extraneous influences of variables commonly associated with behavioral research, representative study design moderators were distinguished from participant characteristics directly pertinent to the research questions. Study design characteristics comprised: (a) cultural context, to account for the various countries in which included studies were conducted; (b) gender balance, because of conflicting information about gender differences in phonological development, [77, 78, 79], (c) sample size, because groups with TD were frequently larger than those with PPD; and (d) literacy evaluation type, due to variation in tests used to measure a given construct.

Directly related to the research questions were the participant moderators, including mean age (within one-year intervals) and characterization of PPD at the point of literacy evaluation. The mean age grouping variable compared early (*learning to read*) with later (*reading to learn*) childhood literacy acquisition whereas characterization of PPD encompassed: (a) resolution, i.e., groups with and without a proportion of children with resolved PPD, (b) severity/subtypes, i.e., moderate to severe, with or without mild PPD), and (c) elicitation contexts (single words versus connected speech, and word length by syllables, i.e., MSWs).

Further to severity/subtypes, those making reference to consistency (*delay, consistent* and *inconsistent*) were coded for infrequently. To increase available sample sizes for testing of moderators, the coders compared descriptions of these subtypes (B. Dodd, personal communication, January 7, 2013) with traditional severity ratings (*mild, moderate, severe*) and agreed to collapse: *delay* with *mild;* and *consistent* and *inconsistent,* with *moderate to severe* and *severe. Child Apraxia of Speech* was also included in the latter group. Bias was considered minimized by: (a) the small number of samples in the *mild* category coded for *delay* (*PA, NWD* and *SP* [n=18]; *DEC* [n=19]); and (b) grouping the *moderate to severe* and *severe* codes in any tests of moderators. Small sample sizes of groups coded with more severe or persistent PPD precluded separate analyses.

RESULTS

The *effect size* data (*Cohen's d*) were examined to address the research questions concerning word level literacy acquisition of children with PPD in comparison to peers with typically developing phonology (TD). In this regard, the descriptive analysis first outlines to what extent children with PPD are disadvantaged in word level literacy. Moderate to large magnitudes of difference were predicted for each literacy construct, with the greatest in *SP*.

Findings pertaining to these predictions will be discussed by construct in the following order: *Phonological Awareness (PA), Word Decoding (DEC), Fluency (FL), Nonword Decoding (NWD)* and *Spelling (SP).*

In the subsequent section concerning inferential results, MRAs of *ESs* and assessment of study design moderators are presented first. Then, the research questions about literacy acquisition in children with and without PPD are addressed. Regarding stage of literacy acquisition, differences were expected in both early and later stages, with larger differences in the later stage, assuming a slower developmental trajectory in children with PPD. [10] The final question addressed potential differences according to the characterization of PPD. [36] A first prediction was that degree of PPD at time of literacy measurement would explain variation in literacy outcomes, whether defined in terms of severity and sub-type, or by resolution. Second, it was predicted that speech evaluation method would also moderate word level literacy outcomes and support the need to assess phonologically complex speech contexts (i.e., MSWs and connected speech) in school-aged children.

Descriptive Analysis Results

Relevant to the descriptive results are the visual displays of data in funnel and forest plots for the *unbiased d* and *mixed weighted ds,* respectively (see Appendices A and B). Data for four literacy constructs, *PA*, *DEC, NWD* and *SP,* are displayed in both plots, but because the sample for *FL* was small (n = 4), only the related forest plot was constructed. The funnel plots depict the distributions of *unbiased d*, from which outliers can be visualized. The treatment of outliers was to adjust *ES* accuracy through weighting by the inverse variance, enabling retention of all data in the statistical analysis. For the *mixed weighted ds* (weighted additionally by the *REVC*), the forest plots convey the *ES* values, the 95% *Confidence Intervals* (*CIs*) of each study and of the mean *d*, with associated 95% *Credibility Intervals* (*CredInts*). The forest plots confirmed moderate to large effect sizes between children with and without PPD on the literacy constructs, as follows: moderate for *DEC* and *NWD* and large for *PA, FL* and *SP*. The means for *PA*, *DEC*, *NWD* and *SP* were significant but only that for *PA* was generalizable to other populations of studies. Further details concerning these findings are reported below.

With reference to the funnel plots for *PA*, *DEC, NWD* and *SP* (Figure A1 to Figure A4, respectively), distributions were normalized using logarithmic lines, setting limits at three standard deviations. In the subsequent assessment of outliers, attention was given to negative values of *unbiased d*, whereby children with PPD outperformed those with TD, a less expected outcome. Negative *ES* outliers were observed in the plots for *DEC* and *NWD* only and were few, specifically: *DEC* = 2 (n = 17); *NWD* = 3 (n = 9). In the raw data for *FL* (n = 4), there was one negative value. However, because the weighting procedures were expected to adjust these values and all other outliers sufficiently, negative outliers were retained in the subsequent analyses. This procedure avoided selective data removal and consequent reduction of construct sample sizes.

The respective forest plots for *PA*, *DEC, NWD*, *SP*, and *FL* are displayed in Figure B1 to Figure B5, respectively, and are referenced below. The forest plots show the range of the *mixed weighted d* for each included study, and the *mean* for the construct, with the interval estimates of significance (95% *CI* and 95% *CredInt*). For *PA,* (see Figure B1) two study *CIs* were without significance; however, the *CI* and *CredInt* indicated a significant large mean (*d* = 0.85; range = -0.02 to 7.90). For *DEC,* (see Figure B2), five study *ds* were not significant but the *CI* suggested a significant moderate mean (*d* = 0.63; range = -1.51 to 4.99). For *NWD* (see Figure B3), three study *ds* were without significance but the *CI* was significant for the moderate mean (*d* = 0.50; range = -1.25 to 3.38). Regarding *SP*, Figure B4 showed nonsignificant *ESs* of four studies but a significant *CI* for the large mean (*d* = 0.84; range = -0.66 to 4.67). For *FL*, Figure B5 demonstrated the significant large *ES* for the study by Puranik et al. (2007) [10]; however, the mean for the construct was not significant (*d* = 3.04; range = -0.005 -0.09).

In summary, for all literacy constructs, predictions of moderate to large differences were substantiated between the mean *mixed weighted ds* for groups with and without PPD. The largest *ES* was predicted for *SP*; however, the largest was found for *FL*, and the *ESs* for *PA* and *SP* were equivalent. In spite of the greater difficulty attributed to *NWD* than *DEC*, a moderate mean effect was obtained for both constructs. Concerning generalization, the mean *mixed weighted d* for the small *FL* sample was without significance. In contrast, the *95% CIs* for all other constructs suggested significant means, but only the *95% CredInt* for *PA* indicated that the *mean ES* was also generalizable to other possible populations.

Inferential Analysis Results

Results for the Multiple Regression Analysis (MRA)

Two separate MRAs were conducted to determine if there was significant variance ($p < .05$) among the *ESs* of any of the constructs to allow testing of moderators. Both a fixed effects model (which assumes that all possible studies were included), and a random effects model (which assumes that the analyzed studies were estimating for different populations) were implemented for the *weighted* and *mixed weighted ds*, respectively.

A theoretical model was constructed that considered the incremental demands on phonological and orthographic knowledge, plus availability of semantic cues. This model was used to establish a hierarchical order for entering a single literacy construct at each step: *PA, DEC, FL, NWD* and *SP*. In the first regression, the R^2 *change* (*ES* for MRA) reached significance once *NWD* was entered, $F(3,60) = 6.17$, $p = .001$. The addition of *SP* also resulted in a significant model, $F(4,60) = 4.55$, $p < .003$; however, the R^2 *change* was not significant, indicating that only *NWD* accounted for the significance of the last two models.

In the second regression of the *mixed weighted ds,* the R^2 *change* for all four models was significant (see Table 1). The constant, *PA*, was also significant, $t = 5.71$, $p < .001$. Therefore, all of *PA, DEC, NWD* and *SP* had additional variance to explain for the moderator analysis. Because the sample size for *FL* was too small to make meaningful comparisons on the moderators, it was not examined further.

Table 1. Model Summary for Multiple Regression of *mixed weighted d* for the Literacy Constructs

Model	*R*	R^2	*Adj* R^2	*Se*	ΔR^2	ΔF	df1	df2	Sig ΔF
*PA*DEC*	.345	0.119	0.105	1.87	0.12	8.35	1	62	0.005
*PA*DEC*FL*	.475	0.226	0.2	1.77	0.11	8.44	1	61	0.005
*PA*DEC*FL*NWD*	.534	0.285	0.249	1.71	0.06	4.96	1	60	0.03
*PA*DEC*FL*NWD*SP*	.842	0.709	0.689	1.10	0.42	85.96	1	59	0

Note. PA = Phonological Awareness. DEC =Word Decoding. NWD = Nonword Decoding. FL = Fluency. SP = Spelling.

Result for the constant, PA: $t = .571$, $p < .001$.

$^*p < .05$.

Results for the Testing of Moderators

The analysis next concerned the significance of the moderators on the *Q*-tests of between-groups variances for the mean *mixed weighted ds* ($p < .05$), first for study design and then participant characteristics. For each literacy construct, these results and those for the *Q*-tests of homogeneity of variances within groups ($p < .05$) are presented in detail in Appendices C to F. Although the intent was to test all literacy constructs (*PA, DEC, NWD* and *SP*) on all moderators, constructs with insufficient samples of *ESs* were excluded from the analysis.

Study design moderators were initially tested aside from the participant characteristics, in order to address selected factors known to influence developmental behavioral research: cultural range, proportion of male participants, sample size and specific literacy measures used. The subsequent sequence of testing participant characteristics concerned differences in literacy outcomes in earlier versus later childhood literacy phases, and characterization of PPD in terms of severity/sub-types or resolution, and level of speech complexity evaluated (single words versus connected speech, and MSWs).

Results for Study Characteristics

Table 2 summarizes the analyses of the study characteristic moderators. These moderators appeared to have minimal influence on the outcomes for the literacy constructs, with some exceptions for *SP*. For this construct, two moderators were significant, i.e., cultural context and measure used.

With regard to the first moderator, cultural context, included studies were primarily from the United States and England, with a limited number from New Zealand, Scotland and Canada. All constructs were tested on cultural context, with nonsignificant results, with the exception of *SP*. For this construct, there were differences between the United States and England, whether or not either country was grouped with New Zealand, Scotland and/or Canada.

The next moderator, gender ratio, was examined to ascertain whether literacy outcomes reflected proportions of girls and boys in the study. Balanced gender was defined as near 50%, but no more than 60% male, to allow latitude for the greater likelihood of protracted speech and language development in boys. The gender moderator was not significant for groups with PPD, and homogeneity was reached on one construct, *SP*.

Regarding groups with TD, gender ratio was balanced in all but one study of *NWD* (n=9), and so was not tested. Of the three remaining constructs (*PA,*

DEC and *SP*), only *PA* was significant, comparing respective large and moderate *ESs* for balanced and unbalanced gender. Unexpectedly, the larger *ES* pertained to groups with smaller as opposed to larger proportions of boys. Considering the small number of *PA* studies lacking gender balance (4 of 18), gender ratio did not appear to have a substantial influence on group literacy differences in the included studies.

Table 2. Study Moderators Tested and Significance across Constructs

Moderator	Groups Tested	*PA*	*DEC*	*NWD*	*SP*
Cultural Context	US vs England (with/without other[a])	✓	✓	✓	*
Proportion Male Participants					
PPD	Near 50% to 60% vs 61 to 70%+	✓	✓	✓	✓
TD	Near 50% to 60% vs 61 to 70%+	*	✓		*
Sample Size					
n_{PPD}	4 to 25 vs 30 to 98	✓	*	*	*
n_{TD}	4 to 44 vs 98 to 815	*	✓	*	*
Measures of Construct[b]	Standardized & Nonstandardized	✓	✓		*
	Specific Standardized		✓		✓

Note. PA = Phonological Awareness. DEC = Word Decoding. NWD = Nonword Decoding. SP = Spelling. PPD = Protracted Phonological Development. TD = Typical Development.

[a]Other = New Zealand, Scotland and/or Canada. [b]Because NWD was typically evaluated with the Woodcock Reading Mastery Tests (WRMT; Woodcock, 1987, 1998), no test of moderator was available.

*$p < .05$.

With respect to the third study design moderator, sample size, significant results would have confirmed the expectation that larger *ESs* are related to larger samples. In the tests of the sample size moderator, comparisons of smaller with larger groups of children (both TD and PPD), reached significance for all constructs, with two exceptions: (a) *PA,* for children with PPD, and (b) *DEC,* for the group with TD.

With respect to children with PPD, across literacy constructs, the mean *weighted ds* for smaller samples ranged from small to moderate but were compared with consistently large *ESs* in larger samples, as expected. Regarding typically developing children, *ESs* were more various; in smaller samples, they ranged from small to large, and were moderate or large in larger samples. However, larger samples of children with and without PPD were related to the largest mean *ds*, as anticipated. Nevertheless, *ESs* in some small studies were possibly underestimating differences between children with and without PPD.

The last study moderator, literacy measure, was tested for differences in construct outcomes from two perspectives on standardization. The first analysis compared evaluations with and without standardization, and the second, specific standardized measures. Non-standardized evaluations were either too small (*DEC, SP*) or too various (*PA*) to be split further. With respect to *NWD*, a particular standardized evaluation, the *Woodcock Reading Mastery Test* (*WRMT*), [59, 60] was the main test used, leaving no meaningful groupings. However, of the differences between standardized and non-standardized measures for *PA, DEC* and *SP*, only *SP* was significant. Large *ESs* were compared on this construct, with the largest ascribed to methods without standardization. This suggested that the types of measures might have been administered differently and/or placed different amounts of emphasis on various orthographic patterns.

Moving to differences among standardized evaluations, comparisons were available for *DEC* and *SP*, with mixed results. In terms of *DEC*, there was no significant difference between measures used within and outside of North America. Conversely, for *SP*, the result was significant between the frequently used *Test of Written Spelling* (*TWS*), [90] and a remaining collection of evaluations. In sum, particular standardized tests did not account for significant variability in literacy outcomes; however, when nonstandardized *SP* measures were used, larger differences were found between children with and without PPD.

Overall, literacy outcomes between children with PPD and typical phonology were not significantly influenced by the study design parameters investigated: cultural range, gender balance, sample size or evaluation method. Exceptions to this concerned *SP,* for which differences were related to countries where studies were conducted (i.e., United States versus England), and to whether or not evaluation methods were standardized.

Results for Participant Characteristics

Turning to participant characteristics, Table 3 summarizes the results for the testing of earlier versus later childhood literacy mean ages, PPD severity and resolution, and level of speech complexity evaluated. Moderators for literacy phase, and PPD characterization were associated with significant differences in *NWD* and *SP* outcomes, while speech complexity had a bearing on all constructs that could be tested, *PA, DEC* and *SP,* as outlined below.

Concerning the first participant moderator, mean age at literacy evaluation, results were significant for *NWD* and *SP* (with adolescent groups removed, e.g., Lewis and Freebairn, 1992 [36]). The test for *SP* also reached homogeneity, suggesting that there was no further variance to explain. Given the caveat of the small sample size for *NWD*, a large *ES* for children in the earlier literacy phase was compared with a negligible mean in the later phase.

Table 3. Participant Moderators Tested and Significance across Constructs

Moderator	Groups Tested	*PA*	*DEC*	*NWD*	*SP*
Range of Mean Age at Literacy[a]	4;0 to 6;11 vs 7;0 to 8:11	✓			
	5;0 to 7;11 vs 8;0 to 10;11		✓	*	*
Resolution	Resolved vs Unresolved	✓	✓	*	*
Severity	Mild & Moderate with/without Severe vs Moderate &/or Severe	✓	✓	*	*
Measures of PPD at Literacy					
Word Lengths	Mono- & Di-syllabic vs Multi- with/without Mono- & Di- syllabic	*	*		*
Speech Context	Single words vs Single words & Connected speech	*	✓		

Note. PA = Phonological Awareness. DEC = Word Decoding. NWD = Nonword Decoding. SP = Spelling. PPD = Protracted Phonological Development. TD = Typical Development.

[a] Closest approximation to earlier and later phases of childhood literacy (Chall,1983).

*$p < .05$

Negligible means were those obtained from two of the three studies of *NWD* in which children with PPD outperformed those with TD. For *SP* and *PA,* the largest *mean weighted d* was also associated with the earlier phase, but moderate *ds* for *DEC* were virtually equivalent. Notwithstanding the incongruity of negative *ESs* for *NWD*, the results indicated greater differences between children with and without PPD in the earlier phase of literacy attainment, but that the range remained moderate to large.

The next tests of moderators concerned characterization of PPD in terms of severity (combined with subtypes) and resolution. Beginning with severity, studies tended to examine ranges from mild to severe, or from moderate to severe, making tests on more discrete categories unavailable. The comparisons these two groups, however, were significant for *NWD* and *SP* but not *PA* and *DEC*. For *NWD*, the group differences were large and negligible, the latter again because of children with PPD out-performing those with TD. For *SP*, significance related to large *mean weighted ds*, in contrast to nonsignificant moderate *ESs* for *PA* and *DEC*. An additional comparison for *PA*, i.e., traditional severity categories versus consistency subtypes, also was not significant, between large *ESs*. Therefore, *SP* appeared set apart from the remaining constructs with regard to moderation by severity category.

The third participant moderator tested, resolution of PPD (i.e., resolved or unresolved), yielded a pattern consistent with that of severity: significant for *NWD* and *SP* but without significance for *PA* and *DEC*. For *NWD* and *DEC*, the resolved group was equally split as to full or mixed resolution, but few were of mixed resolution in the tests for *PA* and *SP*. For *NWD*, *mean ESs* between groups that were unresolved and mixed as to resolution, were large and negligible, respectively. Negative *ESs* in the selected studies accounted for the negligible *ES* of the latter group. For *SP*, large *ESs* were compared, the largest in the unresolved group. Nonsignificant group *ESs* for *PA* were also large but for *DEC*, were moderate.

In summary, whether PPD was characterized in terms of traditional severity categories, consistency subtypes or resolution, results were consistently significant for *SP* and *NWD*, with larger effects in groups with the most protracted development. However, *NWD* comparisons were unique in the proportion of negative *mixed weighted ds* attributed to very small samples (n = 3). In contrast, moderate to large nonsignificant differences for *PA* and *DEC* were maintained between children with PPD and TD.

The last participant moderator regarding characterization of PPD was complexity of speech evaluation context. For this moderator, two tests were possible: single words versus single words combined with connected speech, and in terms of word length by syllables, monosyllabic combined with disyllabic words versus MSWs whether or not combined with mono- and disyllabic words. *PA* and *DEC* were tested with regard to connected speech evaluation, which in the studies was always supplemented with single word assessment. Results were contradictory, with significance for *PA* but not *DEC*. For *PA,* the *ESs* compared were large and moderate, and for *DEC*, both moderate. However, in both cases, the larger *mean* was ascribed to single word evaluation, suggesting that word complexity as opposed to connected speech, was the more relevant context to word level literacy.

Concerning word length differences, *PA, DEC* and *SP* were tested, and all results were significant. *PA* was the only construct for which MSW evaluation could be compared in isolation of shorter words. For this comparison, the difference between large and moderate *mean ESs* was homogeneous, suggesting that the moderator of word length accounted for all of the variance. The tests for *DEC* and *SP* compared moderate and large *mean ESs*, respectively, with the largest effects for studies that included MSW evaluation, whether or not in combination with shorter words. These results also implied that word complexity was a relevant factor in literacy differences.

In summary, the overarching findings of the tests of participant characteristic moderators were threefold. First, the *mean mixed weighted ds* for subgroups remained moderate to large between children with and without PPD on all constructs except *NWD*. This construct, with the smallest sample size, showed an anomalous association with negative *ESs*, suggesting greater caution about the related findings. Second, characterization of PPD in terms of literacy acquisition phase, or severity, as determined by traditional categories (with subtypes included) or resolution, was significant for *NWD* and *SP*, but not *PA* and *DEC*. Irrespective of significance, larger *ESs* were consistently found in groups with the most protracted phonological development. Third, for constructs tested on complexity of speech evaluation context, *PA, DEC* and *SP,* results were significant when MSWs were assessed, whether or not in conjunction with shorter words. A significant result for *PA* when connected speech was combined with single word evaluation, also suggested that the evaluation of short single words alone is insufficient for characterizing the phonology of school-aged children.

DISCUSSION

A meta-analysis was conducted to evaluate contradictory findings in the literature concerning the relationship of protracted phonological development and literacy acquisition. [6, 8, 24] Clarifying the basis for such differences might inform the design of therapies for spoken phonology in the future, which in turn might enhance literacy outcomes. The meta-analysis set out to determine the convergence of evidence about the magnitude of literacy differences, and the moderating effects of central study and participant characteristics.

The meta-analysis examined two possible major sources of variation in literacy outcomes between studies: (1) evaluation of specific word level literacy constructs of *Phonological Awareness (PA), Decoding (DEC), Fluency (FL), Nonword Decoding (NWD)* and *Spelling (SP)*, and (2) participant characteristics regarding age at literacy evaluation and/or characterization of PPD. The ensuing research questions asked whether differences: (a) were consistent across constructs; (b) varied by age in terms of the stage of childhood literacy (earlier, *learning to read*, versus later, *reading to learn*); and (c) varied depending on researchers' characterization of PPD, as defined by severity/subtype, resolution, or the complexity of speech elicitation context (i.e., word length by syllables, or single words versus connected speech). Before answering these questions about participant characteristics, it was necessary to assess whether aspects of study design also explained variance in literacy outcomes; consequently, moderators of cultural context, sample size, gender and specific literacy measures were tested.

Review of Key Methodology for the Meta-analysis

In the next section, the methodology for the meta-analysis is reviewed as a qualifying context for the discussion of descriptive and inferential results that follows.

A descriptive analysis addressed the first question of the study: Are children with PPD consistently disadvantaged in word level literacy acquisition compared with TD peers, and if so, to what extent? Initially, *effect sizes (ESs)* for the mean differences between children with and without PPD (*unbiased Cohen's d*) were calculated for 67 independent samples identified in the 34 included studies. Distributed across the literacy constructs, sample sizes were as follows: *PA* (n = 20), *DEC* (n = 17), *FL* (n = 4), *NWD* (n = 9), and *SP* (n = 14). The *ESs* corresponding to all constructs were predicted to be moderate to large, with the largest expected for *SP*. Outliers were inspected visually in funnel plots. To treat the identified outliers, all *ESs* were weighted by two factors: (a) the *inverse variance*, to adjust study influence by sample size, and (b) the *Random Effects Variance Component* (*REVC*), because the included studies were likely estimating for different populations of studies.

Then, by constructing forest plots of the *95% Confidence Intervals (CIs)* and the 95% *Credibility Intervals (Cred Ints)*, the significance and generalization of *ESs* were examined. The significance of study differences was judged in relation to the *CI* for the construct mean, which also suggested generalization to the population for the sample of included studies. More stringently, the corresponding *Cred Ints* indicated whether the construct mean was representative of all possible populations of studies, completing the descriptive analysis.

An inferential analysis was subsequently conducted to address the primary research questions about participant characteristics. Initially, multiple regression analysis (MRA) was used to establish that there was sufficient variance among the *ESs* on any construct, to test the moderators. The conflicting literacy outcomes identified in the research suggested that all variances would be significant, predictions confirmed by the MRA ($p <.05$). This allowed the moderators of age at literacy measurement and characterization of PPD to be evaluated on the Q statistic (similar to *Chi-square* for categorical variables) whenever constructs had sufficient studies to group on these variables. Following from this requirement, *FL* was excluded from the moderator analyses because of its small sample size.

Before assessing the moderators for the research questions, the study design moderators were tested. Significance was considered possible for cultural context, gender, and specific literacy measures, but less likely for sample size. In terms of cultural context, potential significance related to the range of countries where studies were conducted. Second, concerning gender ratio, a major imbalance was expected to significantly bias *ES* magnitudes in favour of girls. Third, regarding specific literacy measures, moderation could arise from the psychometric rigor of standardized as opposed to non-standardized measures. Further to standardized measures, any differences were predicted to relate to cultural contexts. Finally, with respect to the wide sample size ranges across studies, and between groups with and without PPD, it was expected that the weighting of the *ESs* would be an adequate adjustment.

Following the testing of the study design characteristics, participant characteristics were evaluated in the inferential analysis. Concerning the first of these, age at literacy measurement, it was anticipated that differences between children with and without PPD would have widened by the later childhood literacy phase. Second, the various methods for defining PPD, whether in terms of severity, subtypes or resolution, were all predicted to be significant for two reasons. First, assuming the connection between spoken phonology and word level literacy, [18, 19] more protracted phonological development could reasonably be expected to slow literacy acquisition. Second, it was possible that severity, subtypes and resolution essentially described equivalent constructs of PPD. Last, regarding speech elicitation context, significance was expected because of the added length and complexity of word structure and phoneme sequences in multisyllabic words or connected speech.

Effect Size Results

The first question for the meta-analysis concerned whether differences in word-level literacy skills, between children with and without PPD were consistent. As predicted, uniformity, was demonstrated by moderate to large mean *ESs* between children with and without PPD, for all examined constructs: *PA, DEC, FL, NWD* and *SP*. However, in the examination of outliers, negative *ESs* were unexpectedly identified, indicating that children with PPD had outperformed their typically developing peers. This circumstance bears discussion before further considering the magnitude of the *ESs* overall.

There were two important statistical observations about negative *ESs*: (a) magnitudes were typically negligible, [24, 47] and (b) all were without significance because their *confidence intervals* contained zero. The magnitudes therefore caused little impact on the mean *ES* for a given construct and were not generalizable beyond the primary study. Explanations for the negative direction might relate to several aspects of meta-analytic and primary research methodologies, depending on the construct evaluated. Concerning *PA,* for selected sub-groups with PPD, provision of *PA* intervention [47] could have enhanced performance on dependent *PA* variables. With respect to *DEC, FL* and *NWD*, the meta-analytic calculation of *ESs* from participants' gain on selected data often resulted in a negative value. Consideration of these data, however, showed gain from below average to average-range scores for children with PPD, but from two average range scores for children with typically developing phonology. In some studies, [2, 24, 25] both groups of children lost ground across measurement points, but children with PPD fell behind to a lesser extent. From these observations, it appeared that children with PPD had lower literacy at the outset, and as such, had less to lose.

There were also sample and construct biases in primary studies, unanalyzed in the meta-analytic process, but which may have contributed to negative *ES* findings. Sample bias was probable in terms of: (a) heterogeneous samples stemming from wide age ranges, [36, 64] and (b) children with PPD having higher performance than comparison groups on constructs highly correlated with literacy, e.g., verbal language comprehension and/or production, or nonverbal IQ. [68] Construct validity was relevant to samples that showed equivalent *DEC* and *NWD* attainment in earlier childhood literacy, but that later demonstrated moderate differences in comprehension. [14, 38]

Having considered the influence of negative *ES* outliers, the discussion next deliberates the moderate to large mean *ESs* between children with and without PPD. Such magnitudes were borne out for all constructs examined in word-level literacy; nevertheless, construct-specific magnitudes were not altogether as expected. First, the largest differences were predicted for *SP (mixed weighted d = .84)* because it was theoretically the most complex skill of the included constructs. However, means were also large for *PA (mixed weighted d = .85)* and *FL (mixed weighted d = 3.04).* Next, finding moderate *ESs* for both *DEC (mixed weighted d = .60)* and *NWD (mixed weighted d = .50)* was unanticipated because of suppositions that *NWD* reflects automaticity of sound-symbol relationships. Overall, the *ES* findings suggested that as a group, children with PPD could be expected to score about one standard deviation below peers with TD in *PA* and *SP,* and up to three standard deviations lower in *FL.* For *DEC* and *NWD,* performance of children with PPD appeared approximately one-half of a standard deviation below those with typically developing phonology. Because most studies accounted for SES factors and nonverbal intelligence, the *ESs* derived from the meta-analysis suggested that children with PPD were consistently underachieving in literacy. These differences apparently held *even when children classified as having mild, moderate and severe PPD were examined together (due to inability to isolate sufficient sub-samples in the included studies).*

From a theoretical perspective, explanations for the magnitude of *ESs* found in the current meta-analysis might relate to accessing of phonological and orthographic (i.e., letters) representations. Both types of knowledge are likely utilized to varying degrees from the earliest stages of reading and spelling, [81] with reciprocal influences. [82] Other researchers who shared this perspective, [50, 83, 84, 85, 86] considered phonological representation to be a necessary but insufficient foundation for word decoding. Lehtonen (2009) [82] also argued that beginning knowledge of the relationship of phonemes to alphabetic orthography is required for word-level literacy to emerge. Evidence of other early orthographic knowledge comes from Apel, Wolter and Masterson (2006) [87]. These researchers reported that orthographic processing explained unique variance in young children's spelling detection and written output of novel words, given only minimal exposure to their forms in print. With respect to later literacy, Duncan (2009) [41] defended the notion of ongoing development of phonological and orthographic representations needed to read and spell complex words.

In terms of *ESs* specific to the included literacy constructs, interactions between phonological and orthographic representations that are likely complex lead to relative dependencies that are not uniform. Presumably, speech production is strongly connected to phonological representations that are involved in reading and spelling. Therefore, in tasks of *PA,* primary reliance on phonological organization up until *cracking the code* of print, could account for the large difference between children with and without PPD. As the ability to decode words progresses, reciprocal contributions of the phonological and orthographic systems advance *PA* ability. However, children with history of PPD might continue to be disadvantaged. For example, children might experience confusion over less transparent sound-symbol correspondences, i.e., letters or letter patterns that are associated with more than one speech sound, and the converse, where a single speech sound relates to more than one letter pattern. In another case, children might have difficulty understanding the relationship of a base word to related morphologically complex words. [1]

Mutual dependence on phonological and orthographic representations is more probable for *DEC, FL, NWD* and *SP,* from the outset of their development. Between children with and without PPD, the large *ESs* for *FL* and *SP* could logically be precipitated by the added factor of skill automaticity. Automaticity is required for success in *FL* by definition, [10] but also is relevant to *SP*, [49] because of the overlay of writing the orthography (i.e., insofar as the evaluation methods used in the included studies). Less demand for automaticity could be attributed to the moderate *ESs* pertaining to *DEC* and *NWD*. In both of these processes, speed of connections between phonological and orthographic systems are likely determined by accessing phonological components of assorted sizes, including those related to lexical frequency and neighborhoods, e.g., onset and rime patterns. [41, 82] The lexical restructuring theory suggests that stronger connections to lexical information would facilitate accuracy of *DEC* over *NWD*, [19, 44] in the same way that vocabulary growth is proposed to create ongoing refinement of the spoken phonological system. [88, 89]

A final point of discussion about the mean *ESs* for the literacy constructs concerns generalization. The *95% CIs* were significant for all but *FL*, suggesting that the results for *PA, DEC, NWD* and *SP* were generalizable to other samples of studies described by equivalent moderators. As noted earlier, the very small sample of studies of *FL* (n = 4) and the unique large database sample (n = 10,221) studied by Puranik et al. (2008), [10] made it difficult to draw further conclusions beyond the current included studies. However, the large *ES* calculated from the *FL* data selected for the meta-analysis predicted that *ESs* of similar magnitude could also be expected given similar database samples and *FL* measures. In terms of generalization to populations of studies described by other moderators, only the *95% CredInt* for *PA* was significant, perhaps owing to the breadth of tasks tested that made up the composite scores. The discussion now turns to the assessment of moderators included in the current meta-analysis, first with regard to study characteristics, and then participant characteristics of direct relevance to the remaining research questions.

Study Characteristic Moderators

To explain *ES* differences between children with and without PPD, the literacy outcomes were tested for study moderator influence before addressing the participant characteristics for the main research questions. With the exception of *NWD,* all constructs were tested on cultural context, sample size, gender, and specific literacy measures. *NWD* was excluded from testing on the latter two grouping variables because there were no meaningful splits available. An overall assessment of the results for the study characteristics suggested that effects were not even. However, certain patterns surfaced, including that: (a) gender ratio was primarily not a moderator, (b) sample size was a moderator for several constructs and, (c) effects were more frequent for *SP* than for any other construct. From this general assessment, a more in-depth discussion of the study characteristics selected for the current meta-analysis will first consider cultural context and measure used because of their associations with *SP,* followed by gender and sample size effects.

Concerning *SP,* cultural context and standardization of measures were significant moderators specific to this construct. Cultural context differences were pertinent to the two countries in which the majority of studies took place, the United States and England, but appeared unrelated to differences in particular standardized evaluations. Sub-groups of specific standardized measures compared a more recently published test, the *Test of Written Spelling* (*TWS*), [80] with older publications used outside of the United States, e.g., the

Schonell Graded Word Spelling Test, 1956, [90] and the *Graded Spelling Test*, 1977, [91] also without effect. Therefore, other explanations for cultural differences were considered with regard to spoken English dialect.

Researchers have suggested that it could be useful to confirm whether or not dialect influences skills related to word-level literacy, e.g., morphological awareness. [1] From the perspective of the included studies, differences in American and British spoken English dialects might account for the observed effect of cultural context on *SP*. That is, with regard to sonorous segments (vowels or consonants with spontaneous voicing), spelling challenges might vary because of different pronunciations represented by the same orthography. For example, using tasks of phoneme identification in CVCC and CCVC spellings, Lehtonen (2009) [82] has demonstrated the influence of sonority on *SP*. When sonorant consonants (e.g., *r* and *l*) appeared in consonant clusters in the words (e.g., pl, br, rk, lk), both child and adult speakers of American English more often chunked the consonant with the preceding or following vowel. How speakers of American and British English might treat the same contexts would be of interest, because the dialects contrast as to whether spelled sonorant consonants are pronounced, e.g., *r* or syllabic *l*, in words such as *water* or *bottle*, respectively. School instructional practices in *SP* might also vary accordingly.

Another study characteristic concerning *SP* was the significant effect of non-standardized evaluations, which differed from traditional standard tests that have basal and ceiling effects. For example, Nathan et al. (2004) [32] analyzed the results of British Statutory Assessment Tests that evaluated the spelling of 30 words not normally used in the children's written compositions. Words included both monosyllables and MSWs with and without regular orthographic patterns. Based on whole word scores, children were assigned to one of three academic attainment levels expected for grade in school. However, some studies used methods other than whole word scoring, accounting for spelling of smaller word elements. Snowling and Stackhouse (1983) [31] asked four children identified with *Childhood Apraxia of Speech* to spell 52 familiar CVC words comprised of stop and nasal consonants (i.e., *m, b, p, t, d, n, g* and *k*). Consonant spelling was studied in relation to change across three places of articulation; therefore, vowel spelling was not considered. Apel and Lawrence (2011) [1] scored phonemes and morphemes on a 15-word dictation test. In the latter two studies, relatively large samples of children with and without PPD were examined (i.e., n = 74 and n = 88, respectively), with significant *ESs*. For the group of studies, the significant difference was between large *mean ESs*, but was larger when non-standardized measurement was used. Rather than applying basals and ceilings, it appeared preferable to have children spell a representative sample of word structure and orthographic components [1], thereby gaining a more specific analysis of spelling abilities.

The study characteristic concerning gender ratio, was tested independently in groups with and without PPD for *PA, DEC* and *SP,* and for *NWD,* in the group with PPD. Gender ratio in the group with TD was a moderator for *PA,* but was without significance in any of the other tests. Normative information about childhood phoneme acquisition has sometimes suggested gender differences, [79] but whenever reported, has favoured girls. [91] Therefore, in relation to children with PPD, an effect due to higher male proportions in the group with TD would predictably reduce *ES* differences, a prediction upheld for *PA*. However, other available normative data that have not indicated gender distinctions, [77, 78] were aligned with the nonsignificance of gender ratio in the studies overall.

Sample size was also independently evaluated in groups with and without PPD for all constructs. Sample sizes were often between non-equivalent groups, the largest mainly ascribed to children with TD, [7, 39, 67] because recruiting large samples of participants with PPD is frequently difficult. In the tests of the sample size moderator, only two tests were not significant: children with PPD in studies of *PA*, and those with TD in studies of *DEC*. In the significant comparisons, the largest *mean ES* was attributed to the group of studies with larger samples. Therefore, it is possible that *ESs* were underestimated in the studies with smaller samples of either group of children.

Participant Characteristic Moderators

The discussion moves on to the moderators of central interest in the current meta-analysis, the participant characteristics. These were defined in terms of phase at literacy evaluation, i.e., early (*learning to read*) and later childhood (*reading to learn*), plus parameters characterizing PPD, i.e., severity/sub-types, resolution and complexity of speech context evaluated. In the following section, the results for the tests of each moderator will be discussed in turn and conclude with the support they lend to theoretical views about the course of literacy acquisition for children with PPD.

Regarding age range or phase of literacy development, synopses in the literature offered mixed conclusions about whether there are persistent differences in the literacy of children with and without PPD. [1, 8, 10, 11, 36]

The current meta-analysis suggested ongoing large or moderate differences in *PA, DEC* and *SP*, but not in *NWD*. Also relevant to these differences was whether magnitudes were smaller in the later childhood phase, and any variation in results among the constructs. For *PA* and *DEC,* moderate differences were maintained but in *SP*, differences declined from large to moderate in the later age groups. The *ES* for *NWD* also decreased, from large to negligible, an unexpected finding given that performance of this skill theoretically is highly dependent on the phonological to orthographic relationships of literacy. This unique outcome for *NWD* in the later childhood literacy phase must be considered with caution however. Specifically, the *mean mixed weighted d* was obtained from small samples of children (n = 100) and studies (n = 3), and in two of these, children with PPD outperformed those with TD. Nevertheless, if the difference in *NWD* between children with and without PPD does close by the later phase of childhood literacy, the gain might in turn explain the magnitudes of difference for the other literacy constructs. Researchers have been of the opinion that proficient *NWD* will enable fluent word decoding, [10] and spelling, [49] with reciprocal effects on phonological awareness. [1] Stronger phoneme-to-grapheme correspondences demonstrated in *NWD* should in turn spill over to *SP*. [41] Thus, *SP* proficiency might align with *PA* and *DEC* abilities, as was the case in the current tests of the moderator (i.e., all three constructs with moderate *ESs* in the later phase of childhood literacy). Facility with *NWD* might also have been sufficient to prevent *PA* and *DEC* differences from increasing, enabling some children with PPD to attain word-level literacy in the average range.

Characterization of PPD was also determined to be relevant. The first characteristic examined was the children's status in terms of resolution of PPD. Coding on this parameter generated studies of children whose PPD was unresolved, resolved or mixed (a combination of both). In order to avoid confounding the group of studies of unresolved PPD, studies of mixed samples were added to those that examined children with resolved PPD exclusively. This strategy potentially reduced the *ES* for the group mixed as to resolution of PPD. However, for each literacy construct, the proportion of resolved PPD in the sub-group was always greater (range = 0.67 to 0.80), with relative increases in the mean *ES*. This circumstance helped to minimize the confound.

The tests of the resolution moderator resembled those for age range in two respects: (a) the magnitudes of the sub-group mean *ESs,* and (b) the significance of results. For *PA* and *SP*, the mean *ESs* were large, and for *DEC* were moderate, whereas large and negligible *ESs* were tested for *NWD.* Results were significant for *SP* and *NWD,* but not for *PA* and *DEC*. Whether or not significant, differences between children with PPD and TD were not confined to groups of children with solely unresolved PPD. The results for *NWD* were again exceptional, suggesting that children with resolved PPD history did not differ from children with TD. However, as described above, the small sample of studies of *NWD*, including those in which children with PPD outperformed those with TD, suggested caution in interpreting this outcome.

The differing results among the literacy constructs on the tests of resolution were possibly related to the numerous methods that determined status of PPD, used singly and in combinations. Frequently, percent consonants and/or vowels correct (PCC/PVC) were determined for published elicited single word tests or conversational samples. Criterion-referenced cut-offs were established for these measures in terms of percentile rank, standard score, number of phonological processes, or percentage of whole word production inconsistency. Puranik et al. (2008) [10] also described various Florida Department of Education therapy eligibility criteria that referred to either: number and years of delayed consonants in relation to normative acquisition data, intelligibility judgment, disordered error patterns, or rating of moderate to severe impairment on an articulation rating scale. Nevertheless, the similarity of results for the tests of resolution compared with age at literacy measurement, suggested that both moderators indexed growth in phonology and literacy. Puranik et al. (2008) [10] presented such a trajectory for children with PPD in terms of *FL*, from Grade 1 through Grade 3, with marginal differences indicated between children with persistent as opposed to resolved PPD.

Severity or sub-type categories relative to characterization of PPD were tested in two ways: by comparing traditional severity categories with inconsistency sub-types, and by comparing rankings within severity categories. Sufficient studies existed for testing the inconsistency subtypes only for *PA*, with nonsignificant results. Although limited to *PA*, this outcome supported the validity of combining the subtypes with the traditional severity categories, affording a larger sample size for the second comparison. Within severity categories, tests of moderate to severe and mild PPD were conducted. The magnitudes of sub-group *ESs* for each construct replicated those used in the tests of mean age and resolution, in addition to iterating the patterns of significance, i.e., significant results for *NWD* and *SP* but nonsignificant for *PA* and *DEC*. For all literacy constructs, the analogous results for resolution and severity/subtype categories suggested that the moderators defined equivalent constructs of PPD, and represented the course of the children's phonological development. For some children not identified with PPD until the early phase in which literacy was also evaluated, severity/subtype and resolution coincided. Where children were identified prior to the later phase in which literacy was measured, severity/subtype and resolution measured status of PPD at different points on the continuum.

Specific evaluation methods were also relevant to characterization of PPD. The results of the meta-analysis suggested that a more useful option for understanding the relationships between PPD and literacy was to use continuous rather than categorical levels of measurement, as argued by Peterson et al. (2008). [8] In the current meta-analysis, the appropriate complexity of speech context for obtaining such levels of measurement was tested in terms of evaluation of connected speech and of multisyllabic words in the phonological assessments. Researchers have contended that proficiency of spoken MSWs is relevant to whether PPD is resolved, and in turn, to literacy outcomes, and so MSW evaluation was predicted to be a significant moderator. [3, 9, 36, 37, 47, 53, 58] In comparison with mono- and disyllabic single word elicitation, the additional complexity of spoken phonology in connected speech was also expected to significantly moderate literacy differences. The only construct that could not be tested on the speech complexity moderators was *NWD*, but comparisons on the remaining constructs suggested that context made a difference. Specifically, on the moderator of word length, results were significant for *PA*, *DEC* and *SP* and the connected speech moderator was also significant for *PA*. The significance of these moderators, which differed from the outcomes of resolution and severity/sub-types, might concern sampling of children in the various studies. Children whose phonology had not been assessed in more complex phonological contexts might have been assigned to categories of resolved or less severe PPD, or possibly excluded from studies altogether.

Further to evaluation of word length, MSWs was an important factor, with significant effects on all of the tested constructs, *PA*, *DEC* and *SP*. Results were signficant when evaluation of mono- and disyllabic words was compared with assessment of MSWs with or without mono- and disyllabic words. These findings suggested that the addition of MSWs provided supplemental information about the children's phonological development. For *PA*, the effect of MSW evaluation was further highlighted when studies that had amalgamated mono-, di- and multisyllabic words were removed, resulting in a significant homogeneous comparison of mono- and di-syllables with MSWs. Regarding *ES* magnitudes, the studies that evaluated MSWs showed a large difference between children with and without PPD, whereas the difference was moderate for studies that assessed principally mono- and di-syllables. With respect to *DEC*, moderate *ESs* were tested and for *SP*, *ESs* were large, as opposed to moderate, when more MSWs were evaluated.

The final examination of speech context compared studies that only evaluated single words versus those that combined single words with connected speech. This was considered a valid comparison because assessment of phonology in connected speech generally entails also examining single word elicitations. [34] Of the literacy constructs, only *PA* and *DEC* could be tested on the moderator of connected speech assessment, with *PA* significant and *DEC* not. Concerning *PA*, the magnitudes of the *ESs* in the significant comparison for single words were larger than were tested in the combination of single words and connected speech. In contrast to predictions, this finding suggested that the general structure of words in connected speech might have been simpler than that of elicitation corpora. This is consistent with Shriberg and Morrison (1992), [33] who reported that in comparison with word-elicitation tests, words in conversational samples were simpler in structure, and included a relatively lower proportion of multisyllabic words.

In summary, for the participant characteristics, three patterns were identified. First, *NWD* and *SP* were moderated by all of the participant characteristics, whereas only the evaluation method for PPD had effects on *PA* and *DEC*. These results support suggestions that *NWD* and *SP* are more sensitive to the strength of, or access to underlying phonological representations, possibly because of heavier reliance on systematic connections between phonological and orthographic representations. [49, 55] A second pattern was the significance of PPD assessment methods for all constructs tested, i.e., *PA*, *DEC* and *SP*. Phonological evaluation methods appear to be a crucial variable for differentiating literacy performance of children with and without PPD, and are relevant to a continuous scale of measurement, [8] as opposed to categorization by severity/sub-type or resolution. The third pattern concerned specific contexts of phonological assessment, particularly MSW evaluation. Studies that included these complex phonological contexts during assessment, showed more systematic relationships with literacy acquisition. This has clinical implications, as discussed below in the conclusions.

Theoretical Views about Lower Literacy in Children with PPD

Both uni- and multi-dimensional interpretations have appeared in the literature to explain the relationship of PPD and lower literacy skills. Unidimensional explanations refer either to an underlying cognitive process or to the developmental timeline of child phonology. A cognitive view is that a *core phonological deficit* contributes to poor phonological representations that slow down the acquisition of literacy skills. [85] In terms of the pace of phonological development, supporters of *the critical age hypothesis*, [32] suggest that the impact of PPD on literacy is mitigated significantly by resolution prior to formal literacy instruction. Other recent perspectives have favored the interaction of multiple components in word-level literacy, in terms of: (a) multiple linguistic and nonverbal cognitive deficits, [8, 11] (b) synergies between language-based skills, [36] and (c) overlaps of multiple levels of linguistic awareness, including phonemic, morpho-syntactic and orthographic components. [1, 5] Because the moderating effects of the participant characteristics were various, the current meta-analysis substantiates a version of multiple component interaction for explaining the relationship between PPD and word-level literacy acquisition. To the contrary, consistently significant moderating effects on all of the literacy constructs would have supported a core deficit in phonological representations in children with PPD. Alternatively, no effects in the later literacy phase, nor in terms of reduced severity or resolution, would have defended a critical age by which phonology must be *normalized*. Conceptions about the interaction of multiple linguistic components are more convincing in terms of both current language processing models, [92] and nonlinear linguistic theories of spoken phonology. [27] These explanations were also more consistent with the significant effects of speech production context, particularly with regard to the complexity of MSWs.

CONCLUSION

The current meta-analysis was the first to systematically examine the relationship of PPD and literacy. Moderate to large differences were found between children with and without PPD on all of the word level literacy constructs, and were larger in the earlier than in the later childhood literacy phase. Cultural context (United States versus England) was a moderator of *SP*, likely as a result of differences in English dialect. Among the moderators characterizing PPD, all were significant for *NWD* and *SP*, whereas only evaluation method had effects on *PA* and *DEC*. The assessment of phonology in complex linguistic contexts moderated all literacy constructs tested (*PA*, *DEC* and *SP*), mainly regarding evaluation of MSWs, but assessment of phonology in connected speech was also significant for *PA*.

The meta-analysis was limited by the restricted number of studies that could be included, and the small samples generated for each of the literacy constructs (*PA, DEC, FL, NWD* and *SP*), especially for *FL* and *NWD*. Fewer than 25 samples were identified for any of the examined constructs, and fewer than 10 for *NWD* and *FL*. The findings for *PA* were likely the most robust because of the larger sample of studies. The large differences for *FL* between children with and without PPD were not significant, and the small number of studies excluded this construct from the moderator analyses. However, differences for other constructs were significant, and hence generalizable to the population of the included studies (large differences for *PA* and *SP,* and moderate differences for *DEC* and *NWD*). The differences for *PA, NWD* and *SP* were also generalizable to other possible populations of studies. In the future, additional studies of all chosen literacy constructs are needed, particularly of *NWD* and *FL*. More studies could enhance generalizability of findings through a replication of the meta-analysis that evaluates all constructs on all chosen moderators.

Another limitation relative to the restricted set of studies was the number of moderators tested, done in order to reduce the possibility of Type I errors in the significant *Q-tests*. Testing additional moderators in the future might help account for the heterogeneity within sub-groups, particularly because few tests of the moderators had a homogeneous result. Homogeneity was limited to mean age at literacy evaluation for *PA*, and for *SP*, gender in the PPD group, and characterization of PPD in terms of word length. Because it is difficult to isolate generally protracted language development in the characterization of PPD, in future research, evaluating language development as a moderator could inform the relative effects of language and phonology on literacy [8, 36]. Testing narrower age ranges may uncover more incremental differences in literacy acquisition. For example, for *FL,* Puranik et al. (2008) [10] showed developmental trajectories in age levels from one school grade to another, using growth curve modelling.

Methodologies in the studies included also limit the impact of the meta-analysis. There were, overall, relatively low numbers of children with PPD in the selected studies. Researchers have commonly commented on the challenge of acquiring large enough samples with power to detect differences between children with and without PPD. Within the included studies, two-thirds sampled fewer than 25 children in either of the comparison groups and in the remaining one-third, rarely more than 100 children comprised either group. To address the issue of sample size, investigators have recently turned to secondary data from databases, for retrospective study designs. [7, 10] To design larger prospective studies, primary data might also be retrieved (e.g., from CHILDES). [93] A caution about these alternate methodologies is the inability to ensure equivalence of procedures for selecting participants and gathering data. Therefore, comparing findings from database samples to those in primary studies would be a valuable future endeavour.

Another issue regarding sampling methodology in the selected studies concerns participant characteristics. For the current meta-analysis, studies had insufficient groups of children with moderate to severe PPD, confirming that more studies are needed concerning the literacy of these children. [30] To increase the validity of categorical characterization of PPD and the ability to compare research results, researchers may need to standardize the evaluations and criteria for sub-group assignment. Alternatively, according to researchers such as Peterson et al. (2009), [8] relationships between PPD and literacy could be evaluated on a continuous scale. In this way, power can also be addressed, while avoiding semantic confusion of category labels and the arbitrary nature of participant assignment. Continuous scales could be incorporated in longitudinal designs to better follow the course of PPD and draw conclusions about the strength and direction of the relationships to literacy. Longitudinal designs might further include children with history of PPD whose early childhood literacy seems satisfactory, but whose later literacy is compromised in some way, especially in reading comprehension and written composition. [94]

Another important consideration for evaluating PPD status in future studies, also relevant to clinical practice, is the assessment of competence in complex linguistic contexts, the next topic of discussion. Evaluation of linguistic complexity pertains not only to phonological production in connected speech, [8, 12] but also in multisyllabic words. [35, 36, 38] However, there is no theoretically sound norm-referenced multisyllabic word evaluation method that is easily replicable for single word and connected speech elicitation. In research, words tested have varied, [9, 37, 53] and in some cases, variability of whole word production has been evaluated. [47, 58] Creation of a valid MSW corpus necessarily will entail inclusion of representative word structure and consonant sequences, consideration of word familiarity in terms of cultural and academic contexts, and imageability.

The connection between spoken MSW production and literacy demonstrated by the meta-analysis is of clinical relevance in terms of planning intervention for children with PPD. Researchers in literacy have stressed the need for ongoing elaboration of the underlying structure that supports reading and spelling more complex words. [41] This implies that information gained from parallel evaluations of speaking, phonological awareness, reading and writing of MSWs might allow speech-language pathologists to better tailor therapy programs. For example, beyond whole word scoring, more detailed rubrics have been applied to children's spellings, in order to account for the phonological components of words that have not been represented orthographically. [64] Even without benefit of comparable measures for other word-level literacy constructs (i.e., *PA*, *DEC, FL,* and *NWD*), MSWs selected for speech therapy could also be practiced in meaningful word-level literacy to reinforce connections between phonological, orthographic and semantic components.

A final clinical implication of the meta-analysis is the additional support for early intervention. Larger differences between children with and without PPD were observed in the early childhood as opposed to later childhood literacy phase. Potentially, earlier therapy that contributes to progress in the first phase would catalyze further reduction of later differences. Increases in children's performance in *PA* to average or better levels following early intervention, [5] suggest that similar effects are possible for other word-level literacy constructs.

The studies examined here enabled the current meta-analysis by contributing a body of data concerning the relationship of PPD to word-level literacy. The meta-analysis confirmed that children with PPD are at risk for literacy development.

The findings underline the importance of evaluating PPD in complex linguistic contexts, in order not to miss children who appear to have mastered the basics of spoken phonology but continue to be challenged by greater complexity. Future meta-analyses of larger samples of studies are needed that relate literacy attainment to PPD measured on a continuous metric, and that also examine outcomes of different phonological and literacy interventions in the preschool and early school years.

ACKNOWLEDGMENTS

The authors would like to thank Sarah Blois for completing the coding for reliability, and Dr. Nand Kishor for clarification of meta-analysis procedures. The authors would also like to thank Dr. Jeff A. Small and Dr. Julie J. Masterson for supporting the project as part of the first author's doctoral work. Finally, thanks are extended to Valerie Marshall for valuable assistance with formatting.

APPENDIX A: FUNNEL PLOTS OF LITERACY CONSTRUCT *EFFECT SIZES* (*UNBIASED d*)

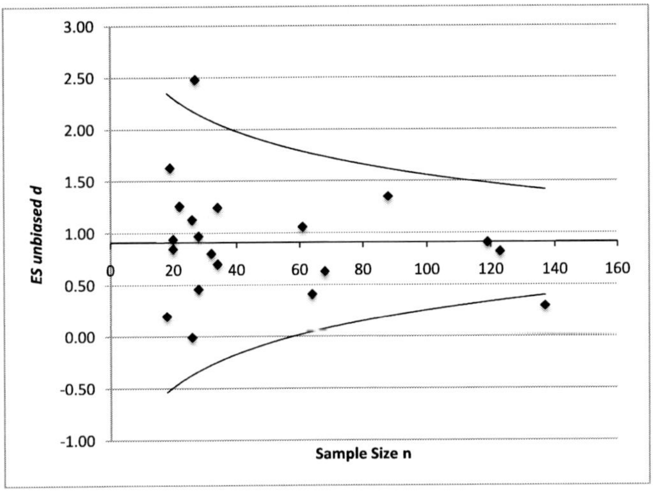

Figure A1. Funnel Plot of *unbiased d* for Phonological Awareness Composites. N = 20.

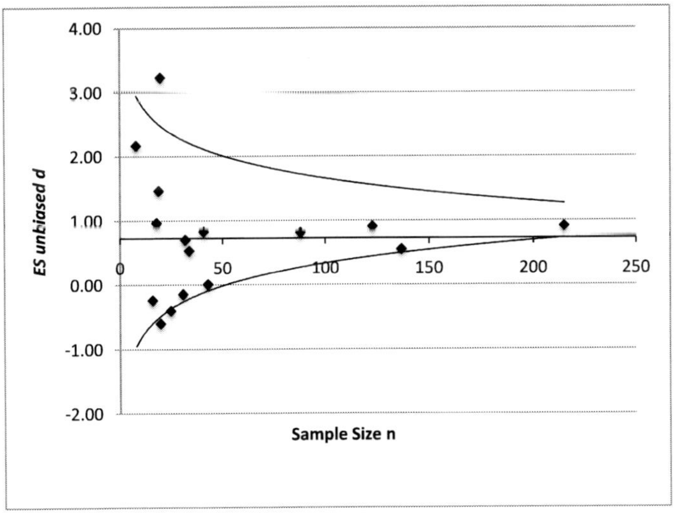

Figure A2. Funnel Plot of *unbiased d* for Word Decoding.
N = 17. Outlier, n = 847; ES = .6704, excluded to expand clustering of smaller n's at bottom of funnel.

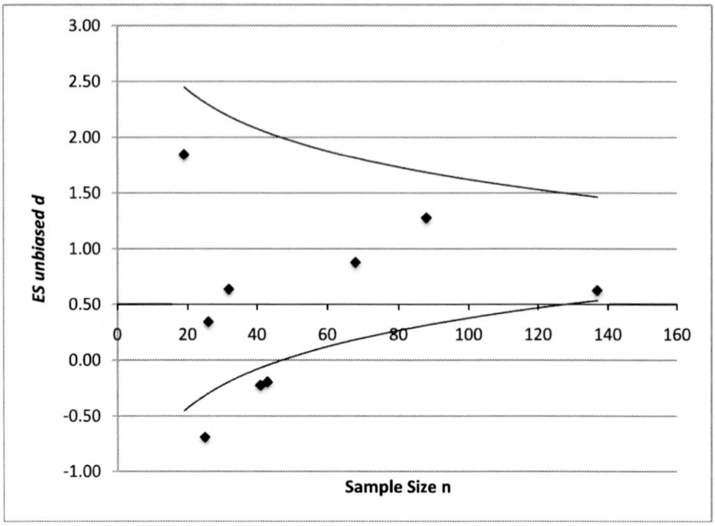

Figure A3. Funnel Plot of *unbiased d* for Nonword Decoding.
N = 9.

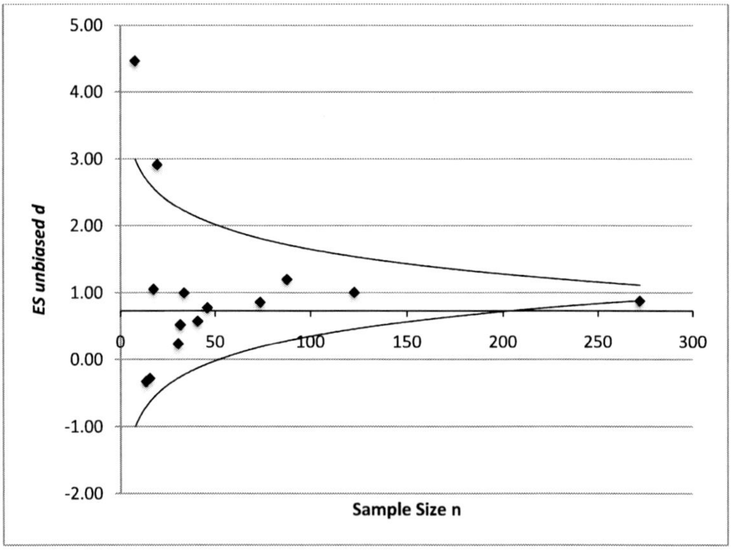

Figure A4. Funnel Plot of *unbiased d* for Spelling.
N = 14.

APPENDIX B: FOREST PLOTS OF LITERACY CONSTRUCT *MIXED WEIGHTED EFFECT SIZES* (d_r^)

	n	d_r^	(95% CI)
McDowell (2004)	137	1.96	(1.19 - 2.72)
Peterson et al., (2009)	123	5.25	(4.47 - 6.02)
Raitano et al. (2004)	119	5.84	(5.06 - 6.61)
Apel & Lawrence (2011)	38	7.90	(7.09 - 8.71)
Rvachew (2007)	58	3.56	(2.74 - 4.38)
Chabon (1980)	54	2.29	(1.46 - 3.12)
Holm et al. (2008[1])	51	4.98	(4.07 - 5.88)
Carroll & Snowling (2004)	34	2.92	(1.96 - 3.88)
Lewis & Freebairn (1992[1])	34	4.88	(3.89 - 5.87)
Meredith (2002)	32	3.15	(2.16 - 4.14)
Webster et al. (1997)	28	1.75	(0.75 - 2.76)
Cowan & Moran (1997)	28	3.53	(2.51 - 4.56)
Preston & Edwards (2007)	27	6.58	(5.37 - 7.78)
Sutherland & Gillon (2007)	26	-0.02	(-1.07 - 1.02)
Rvachew et al. (2003)	26	3.85	(2.79 - 4.91)
Webster & Plante (1992)	22	3.78	(2.65 - 4.92)
Core (2004)	20	2.79	(1.65 - 3.93)
Ekelman (1993)	20	2.54	(1.41 - 3.67)
Harris et al. (2011)	19	3.81	(2.52 - 5.09)
Holm et al. (2008[2])	18	0.58	(-0.56 - 1.72)
Mean		0.85	(0.64 - 1.06)
Credibility Interval			(.19 - 1.51)

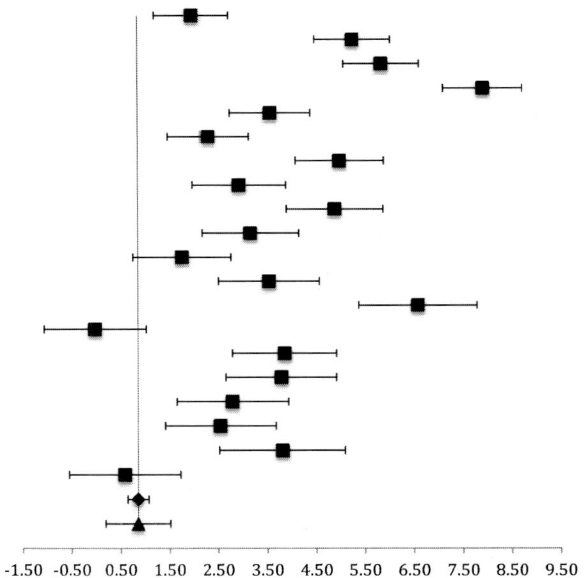

Figure B1. Forest Plot of d_r^ for Phonological Awareness. Random effects model. d_r^ is *unbiased d* weighted by the *inverse variance* and the *Random Effects Variance Component (REVC)*.

Appendix B (continued)

	n	d_r^	(95% CI)
Silva et al. (1984)	847	3.06	(2.14 - 3.97)
Overby et al. (2012)	215	4.27	(3.36 - 5.17)
McDowell (2004)	137	2.49	(1.56 - 3.42)
Peterson et al. (2009)	123	3.98	(3.04 - 4.92)
Apel & Lawrence (2011)	88	3.45	(2.50 - 4.40)
Catts (1993)	43	0.02	(-1.04 - 1.09)
Kirk & Gillon (2003)	41	2.82	(1.75 - 3.88)
Carroll & Snowling (2004)	34	1.74	(0.65 - 2.82)
Meredith (2002)	32	2.18	(1.06 - 3.29)
Bird et al. (1995)	31	-0.45	(-1.56 - 0.66)
Wellman et al. (2011)	25	-0.98	(-2.24 - 0.27)
Ekelman (1993)	20	-1.51	(-2.74 - -0.28)
Stackhouse (1982)	20	4.99	(3.41 - 6.57)
Harris et al. (2011)	19	3.01	(1.64 - 4.38)
Holm et al. (2008[2])	18	2.22	(0.93 - 3.51)
Bishop & Clarkson (2003)	16	-0.54	(-1.85 - 0.76)
Snowling & Stackhouse (1983)	8	2.21	(0.27 - 4.15)
Mean		0.63	(0.36 - 0.90)
Credibility Interval			(-.22 - 1.47)

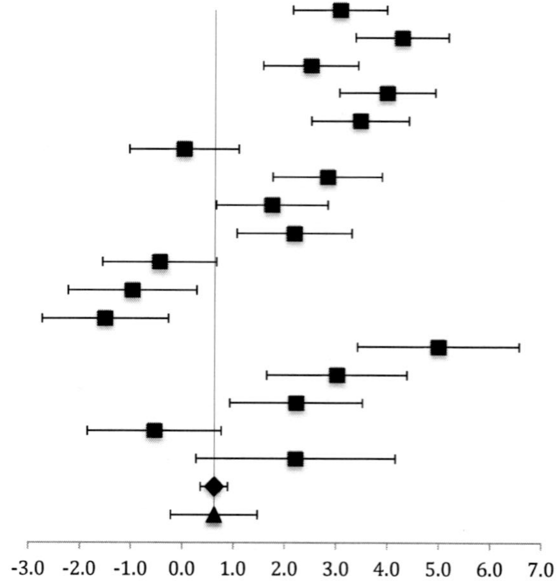

Figure B2. Forest Plot of d_r^ for Word Decoding. Random effects model. d_r^ is *unbiased d* weighted by the inverse variance and the *Random Effects Variance Component (REVC)*.

Appendix B (continued)

	n	d_r^	(95% CI)
McDowell (2004)	137	1.74	(0.56 - 2.92)
Apel & Lawrence (2011)	88	3.38	(2.18 - 4.57)
Rvachew (2007)	68	2.27	(1.05 - 3.5)
Catts (1993)	43	-0.45	(-1.74 - 0.84)
Kirk & Gillon (2003)	41	-0.53	(-1.81 - 0.75)
Meredith (2002)	32	1.39	(0.06 - 2.72)
Sutherland & Gillon (2007)	26	0.69	(-0.70 - 2.07)
Wellman et al. (2011)	25	-1.25	(-2.71 - 0.21)
Harris et al. (2011)	19	2.81	(1.23 - 4.40)
Mean		0.50	(0.06 - 0.93)
Credibility Interval			(-.61 - .61)

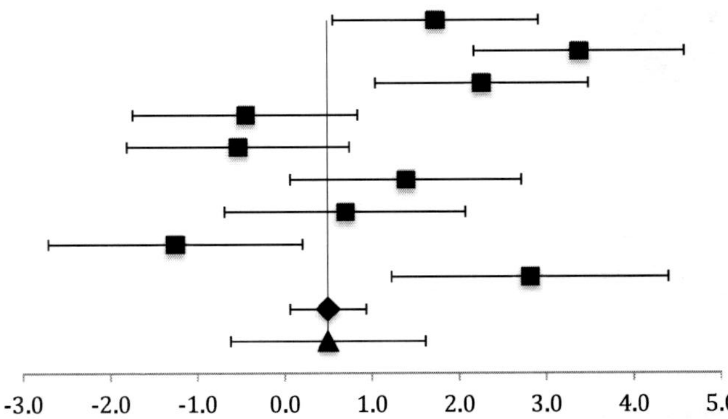

Figure B3. Forest Plot of d_r^ for Nonword Decoding. Random effects model. d_r^ is *unbiased d* weighted by the inverse variance and the *Random Effects Variance Component (REVC)*.

Appendix B (continued)

	n	d_r^	(95% CI)
Overby et al. (2012)	272	3.71	(2.76 - 4.67)
Peterson et al. (2009)	123	3.96	(2.97 - 4.95)
Apel & Lawrence (2011)	88	4.52	(3.52 - 5.53)
Nathan et al. (2004)	74	3.18	(2.16 - 4.20)
Lewis & Freebairn (1992[1])	46	2.55	(1.47 - 3.63)
Kirk & Gillon (2003)	41	1.82	(0.72 - 2.93)
Lewis & Freebairn (1992[2])	34	2.91	(1.76 - 4.06)
Meredith (2002)	32	1.51	(0.36 - 2.67)
Bird et al. (1995)	31	0.69	(-0.46 - 1.84)
Stackhouse (1982)	20	4.67	(3.12 - 6.22)
Holm et al. (2008[2])	18	2.27	(0.93 - 3.60)
Bishop & Clarkson (2003)	16	-0.60	(-1.94 - 0.74)
Burrus (2007)	14	-0.66	(-2.04 - 0.73)
Snowling & Stackhouse (1983)	8	2.28	(-0.46 - 5.02)
Mean		0.84	(0.53 - 1.15)
Credibility Interval			(-.06 - 1.74)

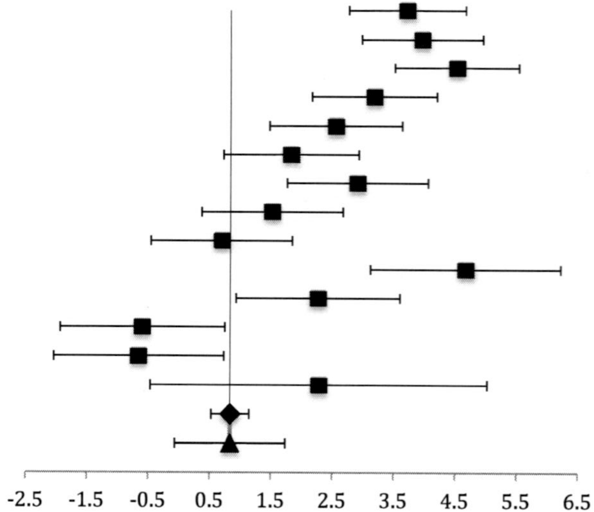

Figure B4. Forest Plot of d_r^ for Spelling. Random effects model; d_r^ is *unbiased d* weighted by the inverse variance and the *Random Effects Variance Component (REVC)*.

Appendix B (continued)

	n	d_r^	(95% CI)	
Puranik et al. (2008)	10221	.09	(.31 - .50)	
Peterson et al. (2009)	123	.006	(-.16 - .18)	
Rvachew (2007)	68	.002	-.48 - .48)	
Catts (1991, 1993)	43	-.005	(-.67 - .66)	
Mean		3.04	(-8.05 - 14.13)	
Credibility Interval			(-19.13 - 25.21)	

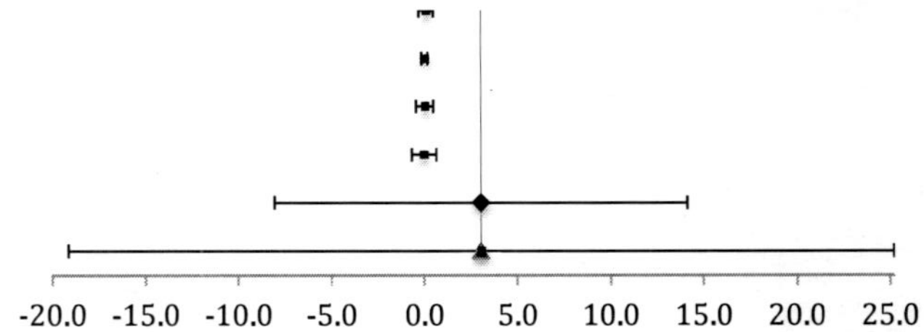

Figure B5. Forest Plot d_r^ for Fluency. Random effects model; d_r^ is *unbiased d* weighted by the inverse variance and the *Random Effects Variance Component (REVC)*.

Appendix C: Results of Tests of Moderators for Phonological Awareness (N = 20)

Study Characteristics						
Moderator	**Groups Tested**	***Mixed Weighted ES (d_r^)***	**n**	**Test for HOV**	**Q between Groups**	**Q within Groups**
Cultural Context	US vs England and Other[a]	0.83 vs 0.73	13 7	Q(19) = 41.12*	2.67	Q(18) = 38.45*
Proportion Male Participants						
PPD	Near 50% to 60% vs 61% to 70%+	0.78 vs 0.90	9 9	Q(17) = 39.96*	3.14	Q(16) = 36.82*
TD	Near 50% to 60% vs 61% to 70%+	0.87 vs 0.45	14 4	Q(17) = 40.51*	5.85*	Q(16) = 34.67*
Sample Size						
N_{PPD}	9 to 19 vs 32 to 86	0.91 vs 0.75	13 7	Q(19) = 41.12*	3.45	Q(18) = 37.67*
N_{TD}	6 to 17 vs 32 to 98	0.92 vs 0.72	14 6	Q(19) = 41.12*	4.31*	Q(18) = 36.81*

Appendix C (continued)

Study Characteristics (continued)						
Moderator	**Groups Tested**	***Mixed Weighted ES*** **(*d_r*)**	**n**	**Q for HOV**	**Q between Groups**	**Q within Groups**
Measures						
Standardized & Nonstandardized	CTOPP, PAT-2, PIPA vs Nonstandardized	0.78 vs 0.84	10 10	Q(19) = 41.12*	2.48	Q(18) = 38.64*
Participant Characteristics						
Mean Age Range at Literacy[b]	4;0 to 6;11 vs 7;0 to 8;11	0.754 0.751	14 4	Q(17) = 26.66*	.41	Q(16) = 26.25
Resolution	Unresolved vs Resolved with/without Unresolved	0.77 0.83	14 5	Q(18) = 41.12*	2.72	Q(17) = 38.39*
Severity	Mild, Moderate with/without Severe vs Delay, Consistent &/or Inconsistent	0.77 0.95	15 3	Q(17) = 39.59*	2.72	Q(16) = 39.86*

Appendix C (continued)

Participant Characteristics (continued)						
Moderator	**Groups Tested**	***Mixed Weighted ES*** $(d_r\cdot)$	**n**	**Test for HOV**	**Q between Groups**	**Q within Groups**
Complexity of Speech Evaluation						
Word Length	Mono- and disyllabic vs Multi-syllabic with/without mono- and disyllabic	0.84 0.77	7 10	Q(16) = 40.97*	3.22	Q(15) = 37.74
	Mono- and disyllabic with/without multi-syllabic vs Multi-syllabic	0.74 0.95	13 4	Q(16) = 40.97*	3.44	Q(15) = 35.73
Contexts	Single words vs Single words & connected speech	0.91 0.68	14 5	Q(18) = 40.95*	4.85*	Q(17) = 36.10*

Note. HOV = Homogeneity of variance within groups. PPD = Protracted Phonological Disorder. TD = Typical development. *CTOPP* = *Comprehensive Test of Phonological Processing* (Wagner et al., 1999). *PAT-2* = *Phonological Awareness Test-2* (Robertson & Salter, 2007). *PIPA* = *Preschool & Primary Inventory of Phonological Awareness* (Dodd et al., 2003).

[a] Other = New Zealand. [b] Months;years.

*p = .05

Appendix D: Results of Tests of Moderators for Word Decoding (N = 17)

Study Characteristics						
Moderator	**Groups Tested**	***Mixed Weighted ES*** ***(d_r^*)***	**n**	**Test for HOV**	**Q between Groups**	**Q within Groups**
Cultural Context	US vs England and Other[a]	0.65 vs 0.67	8 9	Q(16) = 50.01*	0.81	Q(15) = 49.20*
Proportion Male Participants						
PPD	Near 50% to 60% vs 61% to 70%+	0.66 vs 0.76	6 8	Q(13) = 39.18*	0.74	Q(12) = 38.44*
TD	Near 50% to 60% vs 61% to 70%+	0.69 vs 0.83	10 4	Q(13) = 39.18*	0.63*	Q(12) = 38.56*
Sample Size						
N_{PPD}	4 to 19 vs 32 to 86	0.45 vs 0.78	12 5	Q(16) = 50.01*	5.53*	Q(13) = 44.48*
n_{TD}	4 to 44 vs 98 to 815	0.62 vs 0.73	14 3	Q(16) = 50.01*	1.42*	Q(15) = 48.59*

Appendix D (continued)

Study Characteristics (continued)						
Moderator	**Groups Tested**	***Mixed Weighted ES*** **(d_r^)**	**n**	**Test for HOV**	**Q between Groups**	**Q within Groups**
Measures						
Standardized & Nonstandardized	WIAT, WRMT vs Other Standardized and Nonstandardized	0.63 vs 0.73	7 10	Q(16) = 50.01*	1.22	Q(15) = 48.80*
Standardized	WIAT, WRMT vs Other Standardized	0.63 vs 0.69	7 7	Q(13) = 44.92*	0.96	Q(12) = 43.96*
Participant Characteristics						
Mean Age Range at Literacy[b]	5;0 to 7;11 vs 8;0 to 10;11	0.70 0.51	10 7	Q(16) = 50.01*	1.71	Q(15) = 48.30*
Resolution	Unresolved vs Resolved with/without Unresolved	0.73 0.51	11 6	Q(16) = 50.01*	2.84	Q(15) = 47.17*
Severity	Mild, Moderate with/without Severe vs Moderate and/or Severe	0.69 0.62	10 5	Q(14) = 27.47*	.27	Q(13) = 27.20*

Appendix D (continued)

Participant Characteristics (continued)						
Moderator	**Groups Tested**	***Mixed Weighted ES*** $(d_r\hat{})$	**n**	**Test for HOV**	**Q between Groups**	**Q within Groups**
Complexity of Speech Evaluation						
Word Length	Mono- and disyllabic vs Multi-syllabic with/without monosyllabic	0.59 0.73	8 6	Q(13) = 30.24*	4.14*	Q(12) = 26.10*
Contexts	Single words vs Single words & connected speech	0.68 0.63	10 4	Q(13) = 30.24*	3.31*	Q(12) = 26.93*

Note. HOV = Homogeneity of variance within groups. PPD = Protracted Phonological Disorder. TD = Typical development. *WIAT* = *Wechsler Individual Achievement Tests* (Wechsler, 1992a). *WRMT* = *Woodcock Reading Mastery Test* (Woodcock, 1973, 1987, 1998). *TWS* = *Test of Word Spelling* (Larsen et al., 1999).

[a] Other = New Zealand. [b] Months; years.

*p = .05

Appendix E: Results of Tests of Moderators for Nonword Decoding (N = 9)

Moderator	Groups Tested	*Mixed Weighted ES* ($d_r^{\hat{}}$)	n	Test for HOV	Q between Groups	Q within Groups
Study Characteristics						
Cultural Context	US vs England and Other[a]	0.61 vs 0.28	5 3	Q(7) = 34.71*	3.38	Q(6) = 31.33*
Proportion Male Participants						
PPD	Near 50% to 60% vs 61% to 70%+	0.75 vs 0.38	3 4	Q(6) = 27.93*	2.77	Q(5) = 25.16*
Sample Size						
N_{PPD}	9 to 19 vs 33 to 44	0.13 vs 0.89	6 3	Q(8) = 35.20*	14.43*	Q(7) = 20.77*
n_{TD}	6 to 24 vs 30 to 98	0.23 vs 0.75	5 4	Q(8) = 35.20*	6.48*	Q(7) = 28.73*
Participant Characteristics						
Mean Age Range at Literacy[b]	4;0 to 7;11 vs 8;0 to 10;11	0.88 -0.03	5 3	Q(7) = 28.88*	14.21*	Q(6) = 14.67*

Appendix E (continued)

Participant Characteristics (continued)						
Moderator	**Groups Tested**	***Mixed Weighted ES*** ***(d_r^)***	**n**	**Test for HOV**	**Q between Groups**	**Q within Groups**
Resolution	Unresolved vs Resolved	0.88 -0.08	5 4	Q(8) = 35.20*	20.35*	Q(7) = 14.85*
Severity	Mild, Moderate with/without Severe vs Moderate and/or Severe	0.78 -0.16	3 6	Q(8) = 35.20*	15.00*	Q(7) = 20.20*
Complexity of Speech Evaluation						
Word Length	Mono- and disyllabic vs Mono-, di- and multi-syllabic	0.63 0.68	5 3	Q(7) = 26.90*	.07	Q(6) = 26.83*

Note. HOV = Homogeneity of variance within groups. PPD = Protracted Phonological Disorder. TD = Typical development.
[a] Other = New Zealand. [b] Months; years.
* p = .05.

APPENDIX F: RESULTS OF TESTS OF MODERATORS FOR SPELLING (N = 14)

Study Characteristics						
Moderator	**Groups Tested**	***Mixed Weighted ES (d_r^)***	**n**	**Test for HOV**	**Q between Groups**	**Q within Groups**
Cultural Context	US vs England and Other[a]	0.90 vs 0.77	7 7	Q(12) = 41.66*	6.98*	Q(12) = 34.71*
Proportion Male Participants						
PPD	Near 50% to 60% vs 61% to 70%+	0.99 vs 0.85	3 8	Q(10) = 18.97*	2.16	Q(9) = 16.81
TD	Near 50% to 60% vs 61% to 70%+	0.90 vs 0.82	6 6	Q(11) = 22.92*	2.07	Q(10) = 20.86*
Sample Size						
N_{PPD}	4 to 23 vs 39 to 86	0.68 vs 0.97	10 4	Q(13) = 41.69*	9.50*	Q(12) = 32.19*
n_{TD}	4 to 24 vs 35 to 219	0.68 vs 0.97	10 4	Q(13) = 41.69*	9.50*	Q(12) = 32.19*
Measures						
Standardized & Nonstandardized	WIAT, TWS and Other[b] vs Nonstandardized	0.81 vs 0.99	10 4	Q(13) = 41.69*	7.47*	Q(12) = 34.22*

Appendix F (continued)

Study Characteristics (continued)						
Moderator	Groups Tested	Mixed Weighted ES (dr^)	n	Test for HOV	Q between Groups	Q within Groups
Measures (continued)						
Standardized only	TWS vs Other[b]	0.64 vs 0.82	4 5	Q(8) = 23.40*	.60	Q(7) = 22.80*
Participant Characteristics						
Mean Age Range at Literacy[c]	5;0 to 7;11 vs 8;0 to10;11	0.94 0.77	5 8	Q(12) = 41.97*	8.00*	Q(11) = 34.00*
Resolution	Unresolved vs Resolved	0.94 0.77	7 6	Q(12) = 41.91*	7.65*	Q(11) = 34.26*
Severity	Mild, Moderate with/without Severe vs Moderate &/or Severe	0.86 0.84	3 7	Q(9) = 25.16*	5.31*	Q(8) = 19.84*
Complexity of Speech Evaluation						
Word Length	Monosyllabic vs Multi-syllabic with/without mono- and disyllabic	0.79 0.87	7 5	Q(11) = 22.66*	5.66*	Q(10) = 17.00

Note. HOV = Homogeneity of variance within groups. PPD = Protracted Phonological Disorder. TD = Typical development. *WIAT* = *Wechsler Individual Achievement Tests* (Wechsler, 1992a. *TWS* = *Test of Word Spelling* (Larsen et al., 1999).

[a] Other = New Zealand. [b] Other = *Graded Word Spelling Test* (Vernon, 1997), *Schonell Graded Spelling Test* (Schonell & Schonell, 1956) and *Metropolitan Achievement Test* (Durost et al., 1959). [c] Months;years.

* $p = .05$

REFERENCES

References marked with an asterisk indicate studies included in the meta-analysis.

[1] *Apel, K., & Lawrence, J. (2011). Contributions of morphological awareness skills to word-level reading and spelling in first-grade children with and without speech sound disorder. *Journal of Speech, Language, and Hearing Research, 54,* 1312-1327.

[2] *Bird, J., Bishop, D. V., & Freeman, N. H. (1995). Phonological Awareness and Literacy Development in Children with Expressive Phonological Impairments. *Journal of Speech and Hearing Research, 38*, 446-462.

[3] Foy, J. G. & Mann, V. A. (2012). Speech production deficits in early readers: Predictors of risk. *Reading and Writing*. doi 10.1007/s11145-011-9300-4.

[4] *Holm, A., Farrier, F., & Dodd, B. (2008[1, 2]). Phonological awareness, reading accuracy and spelling ability of children with inconsistent phonological disorder. *International Journal of Language and Communication Disorders, 43*, 300-302.

[5] *Kirk, C., & Gillon, G. T. (2007). Longitudinal effects of phonological awareness intervention on morphological awareness in children with speech impairment. *Language, Speech and Hearing Services in Schools, 38*, 342-352.

[6] *Meredith, L. N. (2002). Spelling, reading, and phonological processing abilities of children with histories of phonological disorders. Unpublished dissertation. University of Memphis. Tennessee.

[7] *Overby, M. S., Trainin, G., Smit, A. B., Bernthal, J. E., & Nelson, R. (2012). Relationships among speech sound perception, speech sound production, and phonological spelling in second grade children. *Language, Speech, and Hearing Services in Schools, 43*, 97-115.

[8] *Peterson, R. L., Pennington, B. F., Shriberg, L., & Boada, R. (2009). What Influences Literacy Outcome in Children with Speech Sound Disorder? *Journal of Speech, Language, and Hearing Research, 52*, 1175-1188.

[9] *Preston, J., & Edwards, M. L. (2007). Phonological processing skills of adolescents with residual speech sound errors. *Language, Speech and Hearing Services in Schools, 38,* 297-308.

[10] *Puranik C. S., Petscher, Y., Al Otaiba, S., Catts, H. W., & Lonigan, C. J. (2008). Development of oral reading fluency in children with speech or language impairments: A growth curve analysis. *Journal of Learning Disabilities, 41,* 545-560.

[11] *Raitano, N. A., Pennington, B. F., Tunick, R. A., Boada, R., & Shriberg, L. D. (2004). Pre-literacy skills of subgroups of children with speech sound disorders. *Journal of Child Psychiatry and Psychology, 45,* 821-835.

[12] *Rvachew, S. (2007). Phonological Processing and Reading in Children with Speech Sound Disorders. *American Journal of Speech-Language Pathology, 16,* 260-270.

[13] *Webster, P. E., Plante, A. S., & Couvillion, L. M. (1997). Phonologic impairment and prereading: update on a longitudinal study. *Journal of Learning Disabilities, 30*, 365-375.

[14] *Wellman, R. L., Lewis, B. A., Freebairn, L.A., Avrich, A. A., Hansen, A. J., & Stein, C.M. (2011). Narrative ability of children with speech sound disorders and the prediction of later literacy skills. *Language, Speech, and Hearing Services in Schools*, 42, 561-579.

[15] Leitao, S. & Fletcher, J. (2004). Literacy outcomes for students with speech impairment: Long-term follow-up. *International Journal of Language and Communication Disorders, 39,* 245-256.

[16] Lewis, B. A., Freebairn, L. A., & Taylor, H. G. (2000a). Academic outcomes in children with histories of speech sound disorders. *Journal of Communication Disorders, 33*, 89-92.

[17] Lewis, B. A., Freebairn, L. A., & Taylor, H. G. (2000b). Follow-up of children with early expressive phonology disorders. *Journal of Learning Disabilities, 33,* 433-445.

[18] Perfetti, C. A., Landi, N., & Oakhill, J. (2005). The acquisition of reading comprehension skill. In M. Snowling & C. Hulme (Eds.), *The Science of Reading: A Handbook (pp. 227-247).* Oxford: Blackwell Publishing.

[19] Wood, C., Wade-Woolley, L., & Holliman, A. J. (2009). Phonological awareness: Beyond phonemes. In C. Wood & V. Connelly (Eds.), *Contemporary Perspectives on Reading and Spelling (pp. 7-23).* New York, NY: Routledge.

[20] Lewis, B. A., Freebairn, L. A., Hansen, A. J., Iyengar, S. K., & Taylor, H. G. (2004). School-Age follow-up of children with Childhood Apraxia of Speech. *Language, Speech and Hearing Services in Schools, 35,* 122-140.

[21] Schuele, C. M. (2004). The impact of developmental speech and language impairments on the acquisition of literacy skills. *Mental Retardation and Developmental Disabilities Research Reviews, 10*, 176-183.

[22] Peterson, R. L., McGrath, L. M., Smith, S. D., & Pennington, B. F. (2007). Neuropsychology and genetics of speech, language, and literacy disorders. *Pediatric Clinics of North America*, *54*, 543-561.

[23] *Catts, H. W. (1991). Early identification of dyslexia: Evidence from a follow-up study of speech-language impaired children. *Annals of Dyslexia, 41,* 163-177.

[24] *Catts, H. W. (1993). The relationship between speech-language impairments and reading disabilities. *Journal of Speech and Hearing Research, 36*, 948-959.

[25] Catts, H. W., Fey, M. E., Tomblin, J. B., & Zhang, X., (2002). A longitudinal investigation of reading outcomes in children with language impairments. *Journal of Speech, Language, and Hearing Research, 45*, 1142-1157.

[26] Larrivee, L. S., & Catts, H. W. (1999). Early reading achievement in children with expressive phonological disorders. *American Journal of Speech-Language Pathology*, *8,* 118-128.

[27] Bernhardt, B. H. & Stemberger, J. P. (1998). *Handbook of Phonological Development.* San Diego, CA: Academic Press.

[28] Shriberg, L. D., & Kwiatkowski, J. (1982). Phonological disorders I: A diagnostic classification system. *Journal of Speech and Hearing Disorders, 47*, 226-241.

[29] Dodd, B., Holm, A., Crosbie, S., & McCormack, P. (2005). Differential diagnosis of phonological disorders. In B. Dodd (Ed.), *Differential Diagnosis and Treatment of Children with Speech Disorder (pp. 44-70).* London: Whurr.

[30] Lewis, B. A. (2007). Short- and long-term outcomes for children with speech sound disorders. Retrieved, March 20, 2007, from www.cllrnet.ca

[31] *Snowling, M. J., & Stackhouse, J. (1983). Spelling performance of children with developmental verbal dyspraxia. *Developmental Medicine and Child Neuropsychology, 25,* 430-437.

[32] *Nathan, L., Stackhouse, J., Goulandris, N., & Snowling, M.J. (2004). Educational consequences of developmental speech disorder: Key Stage 1 National Curriculum Assessment results in English and Mathematics. *British Journal of Educational Psychology, 74,* 173-186.

[33] Shriberg, L. D., & Morrison, J. (1992). Articulation testing versus conversational speech sampling. *Journal of Speech and Hearing Research, 35,* 259-273.

[34] Skahan, S. M., Watson, M., & Lof, G. L. (2007). Speech-language pathologists' assessment practices for children with suspected speech sound disorders: Results of a national survey. *American Journal of Speech-Language Pathology, 16,* 246-259.

[35] James, D. G. H. (2006). Hippopotamus is so hard to say: Children's acquisition of polysyllabic words. Unpublished dissertation. The University of Sydney. Australia.

[36] *Lewis, B. A., & Freebairn, L. A. (1992). Residual effects of preschool phonology disorders in grade school, adolescence and adulthood. *Journal of Speech and Hearing Research, 35,* 819-832.

[37] *Core, C. W. (2004). Phonological Awareness Skills in Kindergarten Children with and without Phonological Impairment. Unpublished dissertation. University of Florida.

[38] *Ekelman, B. L. (1993). Examining the relationships among speech-language and reading skills in children with a history of speech-language or reading disorders. Unpublished dissertation. Case Western Reserve University. Ohio.

[39] *McDowell, K. D. (2004). Examining relations among expressive phonology, phonological processing, and early decoding skills in children. Unpublished dissertation. Florida State University.

[40] Chall, J. (1983). Stages of Reading Development. New York: McGraw-Hill.

[41] Duncan, L. G. (2009). Acquiring complex reading skills: An exploration of disyllabic reading. In C. Wood & V. Connelly (Eds.), *Contemporary Perspectives on Reading and Spelling (pp. 42-58).* New York, NY: Routledge.

[42] Frith, U. (2002). Resolving the paradoxes of dyslexia. In G. Reid and J. Wearmouth (Eds.), *Dyslexia and literacy: theory and practice (pp. 45-68).* West Sussex, UK: John Wiley & Sons.

[43] Hatcher, P. J., Hulme, C., & Snowling, M. J. (2002). The phonological representations hypothesis of dyslexia: From theory to practice. In G. Reid and J. Wearmouth (Eds.), *Dyslexia and Literacy: Theory and Practice (pp. 69-84).* West Sussex, UK: John Wiley & Sons.

[44] Coltheart, M. (2005). Modeling Reading: The Dual-Route Approach. In M. J. Snowling & C. Hulme (Eds.), *The science of reading: A*

handbook. Blackwell handbooks of developmental psychology (pp. 6-23). Malden: Blackwell Publishing.

[45] Romani, C., Olson, A., & Di Betta, A. M. (2005). Spelling disorders. In C. Hulme & M. J. Snowling (Eds), *The Science of Reading: A Handbook (pp. 431-448).* Wiley-Blackwell: London.

[46] *Rvachew, S., Ohberg, A., Grawburg, M., & Heyding, J. (2003). Phonological awareness and phonemic perception in 4-year-old children with delayed expressive phonology skills. *American Journal of Speech-Language Pathology, 12*, 463-471.

[47] *Sutherland, D., & Gillon, G. T. (2006). Development of Phonological Representations and Phonological Awareness in Children with Speech Impairment. *International Journal of Communication Disorders, 42,* 229-250.

[48] Compton, D. L. (2002). The relationships among phonological processing, orthographic processing, and lexical development in children with reading disabilities. *The Journal of Special Education, 35*(4), 201-210.

[49] Ehri, L. C. (1992). Reconceptualizing the development of sight word reading and its relationship to recoding. In P. B. Gough, L. C. Ehri, & R. Treiman (Eds.), *Reading Acquisition (pp. 107-144).* Hillsdale, NJ: Lawrence Erlbaum.

[50] Tunmer, W. E., & Hoover, W. A. (1992). Cognitive and linguistic factors in learning to read. In P. B. Gough, L. C. Ehri, & R. Treiman (Eds.), *Reading Acquisition (pp. 175-214).* Hillside, NJ: Erlbaum.

[51] Lee, C. H. (2007). Phonological activation in multi-syllabic word recognition. *Journal of Psychological Research, 36*, 1-14.

[52] *Chabon, R. S. (1980). A comparison of normal and articulation impaired children's performance on four measures of phonemic awareness. Unpublished dissertation. University of Pittsburgh. Pennsylvania.

[53] *Carroll, J. M., & Snowling, M. J. (2004). Language and phonological skills in children at high risk of reading difficulties. *Journal of Psychology and Psychiatry: 45,* 631-640.

[54] Bowey, J. A. (2005). Predicting Individual Differences in Learning to Read. In M. J. Snowling & C. Hulme (Eds.), *The science of reading: A handbook. Blackwell handbooks of developmental psychology (pp. 155-172).* Malden: Blackwell Publishing.

[55] Ehri, L. C. (2005). Development of sight word reading: Phases and findings. In M. J. Snowling & C. Hulme (Eds.), *The science of reading:*

A handbook. Blackwell handbooks of developmental psychology (pp. 135-154). Malden: Blackwell Publishing.

[56] Hester, E. & Hodson, B. (2004). The role of phonological representation in decoding skills of young readers. *Child Language Teaching and Therapy, 20*, 115-133.

[57] O'Connor, R. E., Bell, K., Harty, K., Kappel, L., & Sackor, S. (2000). *The Influence of Text Difficulty on Children's Reading Comprehension Growth.* Paper presented at the Annual Meeting of the American Educational Research Association. New Orleans, LA.

[58] *Harris, J., Botting, N., Myers, L., & Dodd, B. (2011). The relationship between speech impairment, phonological awareness and early literacy development. *Australian Journal of Learning Disabilities, 16,* 111-125.

[59] Woodcock, R. W. (1987, 1998). *Woodcock Reading Mastery Tests (WRMT).* Circle Pines, MN: American Guidance Service.

[60] Woodcock, R. W., & Johnson, M. E. B. (1977). *Woodcock-Johnson Tests of Achievement (W-JTA).* Itasca, IL: Riverside.

[61] Kemp, N. (2009). The acquisition of spelling patterns: Early, late or never? In Wood, C. & Connelly, V. (Eds.) *Contemporary Perspectives on Reading and Spelling (pp. 76-92).* New York, NY: Routledge.

[62] Norton, E. S., Kovelman, I., & Petitto, L. (2007). Are there separate neural systems for spelling? New insights into the role of rules and memory in spelling from functional magnetic resonance imaging. *Mind, Brain, and Education, 1,* 48–59.

[63] Critten, S., & Pine, K. J. (2009). Viewing spelling in a cognitive context: Underlying representations and processes. In C. Wood & V. Connelly (Eds.), *Contemporary Perspectives on Reading and Spelling (pp. 92-108).* New York, NY: Routledge.

[64] *Burrus, M. (2007). Spelling skills in children with phonological disorders. Unpublished manuscript. Missouri State University.

[65] *Stackhouse, J. (1982). An investigation of reading and spelling performance in speech disordered children. *British Journal of Disorders of Communication, 17,* 53-60.

[66] *Cowan, W. E. & Moran, M. J. (1997). Phonological awareness skills of children with articulation disorders in Kindergarten to Third Grade. *Journal of Children's Communication Development, 18,* 31-38.

[67] *Silva, P. A., Justin, C., McGee, R., & Williams, S. M. (1984). Some developmental and behavioural characteristics of seven-year-old children with delayed speech development. *British Journal of Disorders of Communication, 19*, 147-154.

[68] *Bishop, D. V. M., & Clarkson, B. (2003). Written language as a window into residual language deficits: A study of children with persistent and residual speech and language impairments. *Cortex, 39,* 215-237.

[69] Hedges, L. V., & Olkin, I. (1985). *Statistical Methods for Meta-Analysis*. New York: Academic Press.

[70] Lipsey, M. W., & Wilson, D. B. (2000). *Practical Meta-analysis.* Thousand Oaks, CA: Sage.

[71] Rosenthal, R. (1991). *Meta-analytic Procedures for Social Research.* CA: Sage.

[72] Catts, H. W. (1986). Speech production/phonological deficits in reading-disordered children. *Journal of Learning Disabilities, 19,* 504-508.

[73] Goldman, R., & Fristoe, M. (1969, 1986). *The Goldman Fristoe Test of Articulation (GFTA).* Circle Pines, MN: American Guidance Service.

[74] Cohen, J., Cohen, P., West, G. S., & Aiken, L. S. (2003). *Applied Multiple Regression/Correlation Analysis for the Behavioral Sciences.* Mahwah, NJ: Lawrence Erlbaum.

[75] Hunter, J. S., & Schmidt, F. L. (1990). *Methods of Meta-analysis: Correcting Error and Bias in Research Findings.* Newbury Park, CA: Sage.

[76] Cohen, J. (1988). *Statistical Power Analysis for the Behavioral Sciences* (2nd ed.). Mahwah, NJ: Lawrence Erlbaum.

[77] Sander, E. (1972). When are speech sounds learned? *Journal of Speech and Hearing Disorders, 37,* 55-63.

[78] Shriberg, L. D., Austin, D., Lewis, B. A., McSweeny, J., & Wilson, D. L. (1997). The Speech Disorders Classification System (SDCS): Extensions and life span reference data. *Journal of Speech, Language and Hearing Research, 40,* 708-722.

[79] Smit, A. B., Hand, L., Freilinger, J. J., Bernthal, J. E., & Bird, A. (1990). The Iowa articulation norms project and its Nebraska replication. *Journal of Speech and Hearing Disorders, 55, 779-798.*

[80] Larsen, S. C., Hammill, D. D., & Moats, L. C. (1999). *Test of Written Spelling-4 (TWS-4).* Austin, TX: Pro-Ed.

[81] Babayağit, S. (2009). Reading and spelling development in transparent alphabetic orthographies: Points of convergence, divergence and arising issues. In C. Wood & V. Connelly (Eds.), *Contemporary Perspectives on Reading and Spelling (pp. 133-148).* New York, NY: Routledge.

[82] Lehtonen, A. (2009). How do children and adults conceptualize phoneme-letter relationships? In C. Wood & V. Connelly (Eds.), *Contemporary Perspectives on Reading and Spelling (pp. 149-167).* New York, NY: Routledge.

[83] Blachman, B. (2000). Phonological awareness. In M. L. Kamil, P. B. Mosenthal, P. D. Pearson, & R. Barr (Eds.), *Handbook of Reading Research: Volume III (pp. 483-502).* Mahwah, NJ: Erlbaum.

[84] McDougall, S., & Hulme, C. (1994). Short-term memory, speech rate and phonological awareness as predictors of learning to read. In C. Hulme & M. Snowling (Eds.) *Reading Development and Dyslexia (pp. 31-44).* Philadelphia, PA: Whurr.

[85] Muter, V. (1994). The influence of phonological awareness and letter knowledge on beginning reading and spelling development. In C. Hulme & M. Snowling (Eds.) *Reading Development and Dyslexia (pp. 45-62).* Philadelphia, PA: Whurr.

[86] Stanovich, K. E. (1992). Speculations on the causes and consequences of individual differences in early reading acquisition. In P. B. Gough, L. C. Ehri, & R. Treiman, *Reading Acquisition (pp. 307-342).* Hillside, NJ: Erlbaum.

[87] Apel, K., Wolter, J. A., & Masterson, J. J. (2006). Effects of phonotactic and orthotactic probabilities during fast mapping on 5-year-olds' learning to spell. *Developmental Neuropsychology*, *29*(1), 21-42.

[88] Rvachew, S. & Brosseau-Lapre, F. (2012). *Developmental Phonological Disorders: Foundations of Clinical Practice.* San Diego, CA: Plural Publishing.

[89] Stoel-Gammon, C. (2011). Relationships between lexical and phonological development in young children. *Journal of Child Language, 38,* 1 34.

[90] Schonell, F., & Schonell, F. (1956). *Diagnostic and Attainment Testing: Including a Manual of Tests, Their Nature, Use, Recording and Interpretation.* London: Oliver& Boyd.

[91] McLeod, S. (2009). Speech sound acquisition. In J. E. Bernthal, N. W. Bankson, & P. Flipsen Jr (Eds.), *Articulation and Phonological disorders: Speech Sound Disorders in Children (pp. 63-119).* Boston, MA: Pearson Education Inc.

[92] Stemberger, J. P. (1992). A connectionist view of child phonology: Phonological processing without phonological processes. In C. A. Ferguson, L. Menn & C. Stoel-Gammon (Eds.), *Phonological*

Development, Models, Research, Implications (pp. 165-190). Timonium, MD: York Press.

[93] MacWhinney, B. (2000). The CHILDES Project: Tools for analyzing talk. 3rd Edition. Vol. 2: The Database. Mahwah, NJ: Lawrence Erlbaum Associates.

[94] Lipka, O., Lesaux, N. K., & Siegel, L. S. (2006). Retrospective analyses of the reading development of grade four students with reading disabilities: Risk status and profiles over 5 years. *Journal of Learning Disabilities, 39*, 364-378.

[95] *Webster, P. E., & Plante, A. S. (1992). Effects of Phonological Impairment on Word, Syllable, and Phoneme Segmentation and Reading. *Language, Speech, and Hearing Services in Schools, 23,* 176-182.

In: Speech, Language and Voice Pathology ISBN: 978-1-63321-958-8
Editor: Pablo Antonio Ysunza

Chapter 6

CLINICAL OUTCOMES IN MEDICAL SPEECH-LANGUAGE PATHOLOGY

Richard M. Merson [*]
and Michael I. Rolnick
Department of Speech and Language Pathology.
Beaumont Health System. Royal Oak, MI, US

ABSTRACT

This chapter will report on a large patient population (est. 20,000 from 1992-2013) from the Beaumont Health System (Michigan) which had been tracked consecutively on two different clinical outcome programs since 1992. The population includes inpatients and outpatients treated at multiple hospital and rehabilitation centers. Adults and children with communication disorders were tracked utilizing a customized clinical outcome software program (The Beaumont Outcome Software System ©, BOSS) with a large clinician based staff. After ten years the Speech-Language Pathology Department , Beaumont Health System transferred their outcome program to the American Speech-Language Hearing Association's National Outcome Measurement System ©, NOMS). This chapter reports and compares the two clinical outcome systems (BOSS© and NOMS©) and discusses how outcome data contributes to Speech-Language Pathology management.

[*] Contact: rickmerson@beaumont.edu

Keywords: Speech, Language, Outcome, Pathology

PURPOSE AND VALUE OF A CLINICAL OUTCOMES

There are many forms of clinical measurement. [1, 2, 3] The scientific development of standardized testing is a long and rigorous process that may include instrumental or psychosocial assessment. Normative standards of disease and management in clinical medicine and rehabilitation are abundant and utilized by clinicians, researchers and academics. These highly sensitive objective measures assist the professional in differential diagnosis, assessing impairment severity and making predictions for future quality of life considerations.[3] Clinical outcomes, however, are functional measures of change overtime on a standardized subjective clinical scale among individuals with a common diagnosis. [2, 4, 5, 6] They are not indications of diagnosis, impairment, absolute performance, competence or capacity. They are poor predictors of the future quality of life or final achievement of rehabilitation potential. They are expressions of progress. They are not highly sensitive, precise measures of overall clinical competence. Nor do they predict permanence. Clinical outcomes can describe the effectiveness of the treatment strategy implemented to improve the patient's status during the time measured. They may be correlated to costs, can be used to compare clinician performance, program types, and analyze patient demographics. They are at the least, a poor predictor of the final possible outcome and at the most an indication of the effectiveness of the treatment intervention at the time. They are a measure of movement, much like a thermostat, that tells nothing about the source, or the future of temperature change, just that there is more or less heat. Outcomes are not like a complex computer program differentially diagnosing diseases, or proposing strategies for treatment programs. Outcomes can tell you there is change and it's moving in the right direction. This is in fact what our payors, administrators, politicians, and patients want to know from our clinical interventions. Center for Medicare-Medicaid System (CMS) does not necessarily want to know the exact outcome or exact achievement but rather the effectiveness of a treatment program to produce progress. [7] That's what they will pay for, and that is what we can describe as "clinical value". Payors, patients and politicians know that the actual outcome is highly dependent on a large series of variables dependent on the individual and environ. They want to pay for progress, and they want a report card compared (benchmarked) with other providers. [6]

Beaumont Outcome Software System© 1995

In the early 1990's William Beaumont Hospital, a 1000 bed multiple hospital and rehabilitation center system decided to take clinical outcomes seriously. Their major departments were encouraged to seek out or develop a system of reporting treatment effectiveness as outcome measures that could be used by program planners, patients, third party payers and professional associations for potential benchmarking. The Speech-Language Pathology Department at Beaumont, began to develop their own computer based entry and analysis system known as the Beaumont Outcome Software System© (BOSS) [8]. The BOSS developed a series of seven point subjective and objective scales (i.e 60 scales for adults and children) used to record severity before and after treatment as judged by clinicians. (Appendix II) The intent was to report treatment effectiveness or clinical progress from the time of admission (initial evaluation) to the discharge from treatment. A very friendly computer form of fifteen patient features was developed to enter into the software database. A more sophisticated software (BOSS©, Fred Weiner, PhD) program was developed to analyze the interactive effects of the patient features (i.e. Admission Score & Date, Discharge Score & Date, Age, Gender, Communication Diagnosis, Clinician, Length of Stay, Number of Clinical Procedures, Charges). [8] A software program was developed for retail distribution and an interface program was developed to allow clinicians to directly enter their BOSS scores on the hospital medical records system. The BOSS was used in our department for eleven years (1995 through 2006) and collected in excess of 20,000 adult and childhood patient outcomes. Our Beaumont Health System has since grown into a 1738 bed multiple medical center organization with a Speech–Language Pathology Department that has over 70 speech-language pathologists providing 60,000 clinical procedures annually. Here is what we discovered.

Grand Average of Clinical Outcomes (1995-2006) at Seven Sites

Table 1 summarizes the BOSS© outcomes from 1995 through 2006. The Beaumont Speech-Language Pathology Department clinical staff (45 clinicians at the time) reported on 20,000 patients discharged from treatment at seven different clinical sites (i.e. (1) Outpatient Voice and Stuttering Clinics,

(2) Center for Children's Speech-Language Disorders, (3) Outpatient Adult Center /Royal Oak, MI, (4) Outpatient Adult Center/Troy. Mi, (5) Inpatient Rehabilitation Unit/ Royal Oak, MI (6) Dysphagia Program /Royal Oak, MI, and (7) Dysphagia Program/ Troy, Mi).

Table 1, illustrates the number (N) of patients treated at each site, the average treatment progress achieved on a 7 point scale at each site, the length of stay in days, the number of procedures (evaluation and treatments) and the average discharge status all on a 7 point scale. Clearly there are variations in these outcomes that reflect the severity and nature of communication disorders. Our Dysphagia Programs average only 7-9 days of treatment with 4-5 treatment sessions and achieve a respectable 5.1 on a scale of 7 ("7" describes a normal swallowing performance). Whereas our Center for Children's Speech-Language Disorders reveals a discharge status of 4.6 with an average of 62 treatment procedures over a period of one year (385 days). The outpatient Voice and Stuttering Clinics average the most progress on a seven point scale (5.7) in 57 days with an average of 3 treatment sessions. The Voice and Stuttering Clinics can be described as clinically efficient, that is greater GAIN for the least COST (i.e. Length of Stay and Number of Treatments). Different communication diagnoses not only require different treatment strategies, involve different length of stay but they also produce different clinical outcomes.

Table 1. Beaumont Outcome Software System © 1995-2006, N: 20,066

Clinic Site	N	Treatment Progress	Length of Stay (days)	Number of Treatments	Discharge Status
Voice & Stu. Clinics	1803	3	57	4.5	5.7
Children's Center	4343	2.4	385	62	4.6
Outpatient Adults/RO	1212	1.2	68.8	23	5.4
Outpatient Adults/Troy	1533	1	59	16	5.3
Inpatient Rehab/RO	1639	1	17	18	5
Dysphagia Program/RO	4197	3.3	9.9	5.1	5.1
Dysphagia Program/Troy	5339	.62	7.1	4.1	5.1
Grand Mean Values		**1.7**	**86.2**	**19**	**5.1**
Total Patients	**20,066**				

Clinical Outcomes (mean values) at Seven Clinical Sites Page 4.

It is valuable to compare our inpatient rehabilitation program (Inpt.Rehab/RO) with our outpatient rehabilitation program, treating similar patients with medical diagnoses of Closed Head Injury, Stroke and other Neuropathologies (i.e Parkinson Disease, Multiple Sclerosis).

The inpatients were treated over a 17 day period and received 18 treatment sessions. They made some progress (1.0 level of movement on a seven point scale) and finished the treatment program at 5.0 (a good discharge scale value).

Compare that to our outpatient adult rehabilitation program where we treated for an average of 68 days (two months) and with 23 treatment sessions and they were discharged at a slightly higher progress level at 5.4. An outpatient program begins treating patients later after their disease onset and those patients can be seen more often with appropriate reimbursement coverage. These patients are shown to make more progress in a longer treatment program. Reaching a level of 5 on the progress scale is what we consider a "functional performance level" Seven would be normal communication skills.

Comparing the two Dysphagia treatment programs in Table 1 it can be noticed that both programs were able to achieve a 5.1 discharge level, which is good functional performance. However the RO Dysphagia program had a longer length of stay (9.9) and greater treatment progress (3.3) with 5.1 procedures. They saw their patients early in the onset of their disability. The TROY program saw them later post-onset and made less progress in fewer days and fewer treatments but still achieved the same Discharge level. The programs were not different in their treatment effect but the patients were seen at different times post-onset.

These grand average clinical outcomes in Table 1 illustrate how different our clinical program strategies need to be to accomplish a good clinical outcome. Some of our programs are considerably more expensive (length of stay or number of procedures) like our Children's Center of Speech – Language Disorders, when compared to our outpatient Voice and Stuttering Clinics or our Dysphagia programs. Nonetheless, all these services are demanded by our medical community, and we usually succeed at getting all our patients to a Discharge level of 5, which is considered a good "functional level of performance".

Average Outcomes of Three Outpatient Clinics in 2000

Table 2 illustrates all the outcomes collected at three very different outpatient sites in 2000.

Table 2. Beaumont Outcome Software System© 2000, Three Sites

Outcome Parameter	Voice & Stuttering	Children's Center	Outpatient Adults
Admission Score	2.74	2.50	4.23
Discharge Score	5.65	4.80	5.28
Clinical Progress	2.9	2.3	1.04
Number of Treatments	4.43	66.6	20.7
Length of Stay	54.1	348.1	64.3
Est.Charges	$515	$4482	$3564
Pt. Satisfaction (7 pt. scale)	6.3	6.7	6.8
N (Completed Treatment)	111 (52%)	185(36%)	81 (83%)
N (Evaluated Only)	214	516	97

Voice & Stuttering Clinics, Children's Center and Outpatient Adult Program Page 5.

The Voice and Stuttering Clinics were at the medical office building (MOB) and you can see that 111 patients of the 214 that were evaluated, completed treatment. That is a 52% of treatment completion rate. Only the patients who completed treatment were used to score outcomes. These patients were initially, moderately severe in their communication disorder outcome rating (admission score 2.7) and were discharged at a 5.6 level which reflects good clinical progress of 2.9 levels. On average they remained in treatment for 54 days and received 4 treatment sessions. This is an extremely efficient (minimal time and good gain) clinical outcome. The shorter the length of stay and the fewer procedures the less the cost to the patient/payor. We estimated on average in circa 2000 year dollars, a total charge of approximately $515.00 for this service. If we compare these outcomes to our Children's Center (BMC) we note comparable admission severity (2.5) with good but less discharge outcome at 4.8 and a very long period of treatment (348 days) with 66 procedures and an estimated 2000 year dollar value of $4482. While we achieve good clinical outcomes with these children it is much costlier to provide these services and achieve the desire outcome. Finally, examining our outpatient adult outcomes (BRHC) we can see that our admission severity level is much less than our Children's Center or our Voice & Stuttering Clinic. These patients have already received inpatient rehabilitation and have made some clinical progress. Their admission severity is 4.2 and they are discharged at a very good 5.3. They required an average of 64 days of treatment and 20 treatment sessions, very likely limited by their insurance caps. The charges in 2000 year dollars was estimated at $3564.00. Different clinical outcome measures (length of stay, number of treatments, and possible reimbursement) can be used to describe different clinical programs.

CHILDREN'S BOSS© OUTCOMES 2000-2006 BY COMMUNICATION DIAGNOSIS

Chart #1, illustrates the different number of treatment procedures required to obtain a good "functional clinical outcome" (5.0 or better) for a particular diagnosis.

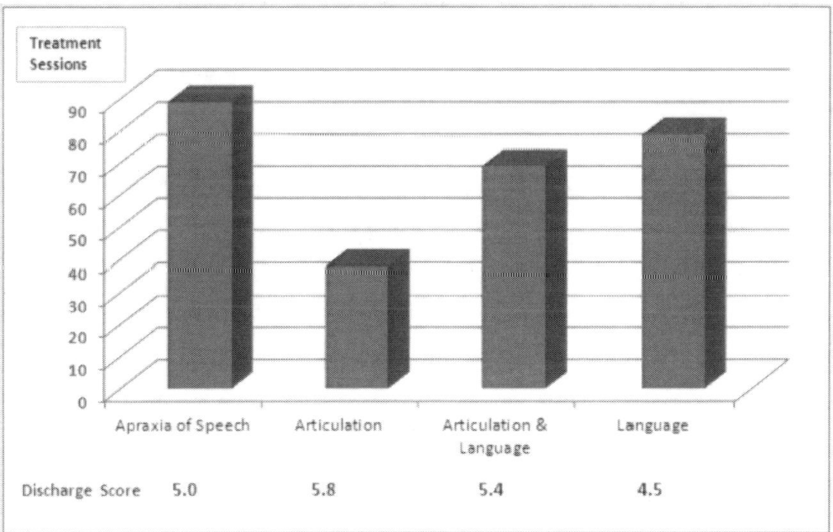

4 Diagnoses by Number of Treatments and Discharge Scores at the Center for Childhood Speech-Language Disorders, Page 6.

Chart 1. Beaumont Outcome Software System © 2000 to 2006, N: 581.

Apraxia of speech in children is a very challenging disorder and in our experience required on average 89 treatment sessions to achieve an outcome of 5.0. Whereas articulation disorders in children required only 38 treatment sessions to obtain a discharge outcome of 5.8, language disorders required more treatment sessions (78) to obtain a discharge score of 4.5. All four childhood communication disorders did well in treatment but each one required a different number of sessions to achieve that outcome. These are important features to discuss with parents when they need to anticipate their costs in keeping their child in a treatment program that is going to have a good outcome.

ADULT BOSS© OUTCOMES IN 2003 BY COMMUNICATION DIAGNOSIS

Table#3, illustrates how different adult communication disorders can exhibit different discharge status outcomes and can require different numbers of treatment sessions and length of stay.

Table 3. Beaumont Outcome Software System© 2003, Adult Outpatients

Communication Diagnosis	Discharge Score	Treatments	Length of Stay	Patient Satisfaction
Aphasia	5.5	19	60	6.4
Apraxia	4.5	15	42	6.2
Dysarthria	5.7	9	29	6.5

3 Adult Communication Diagnoses by Discharge Status, Number of Treatments Length of Stay and Patient Satisfaction. Page 6.

The length of stay (days in treatment) and the number of procedures or treatment sessions can be considered a short hand for the cost to the patient or payor for services. Ideally we want to achieve a positive clinical outcome and leave the patient with a good satisfaction. In Table #3, you can see how treating Aphasia is more time consuming and costlier to the payor/patient than the other diagnoses but we can achieve a very good discharge outcome at 5.5. Apraxia of speech probably had the least effective outcome at 4.5 with 42 treatment sessions. Dysarthria is the least expensive (29 days of treatment) and 9 sessions with an excellent discharge outcome of 5.7. In all three diagnoses, regardless of length of stay or outcome, the patients provided a high satisfaction score (6.4, 6.2 and 6.5).

Clinical Outcomes in Five Comm. Diagnoses in Three Different Years

Sometimes our success with patients can very year to year. In Chart #2, we illustrate how treating the same communication diagnosis in three different years (2000, 2003, 2005) can vary. If we examine Vocal Cord Paralysis patients we notice how the clinical outcome (i.e. amount of progress on a seven point scale) only varied from 3.9 in 2005 to 4.2 in 2003, but in the case of Stuttering the clinical progress varied from 1.0 in 2005 to 3.2 in 2000. The Aphasia group, on the other hand varied very little from .9 to 1.3 to .99 in 2000, 2003 and 2005.

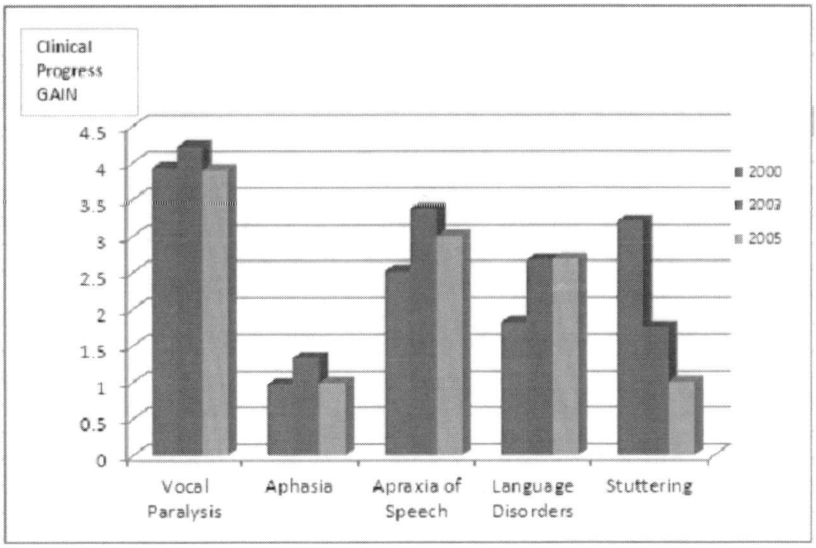

Variations in Discharge Status by Year and Communication Disorder Page 7.

Chart 2. Beaumont Outcome Software System© Variations in Discharge Status.

These variances in GAIN or clinical outcome progress can be attributed to the admission severity level, comorbidities, discontinuance of treatment or motivational issues on the part of these patients. It is interesting to examine the chart and notice how the Aphasia group tends to maintain a lower stereotypic gain in each of the three years sampled compared to the Stuttering group. These differences may be directly related to the complexity of the communication disorder to be treated.

WHAT WE LEARNED FROM THE BEAUMONT OUTCOME SOFTWARE SYSTEM

1. Common discharge GOAL of "5" emerges across all diagnoses by clinicians.
2. Length of stay was predictable and was stereotypic of diagnosis, severity, & complexity.
3. Cost was related to LOS.
4. Referral patterns and comorbidity affected outcomes. Early referrals better, late and re-admits worse. Less comorbidity resulted in better outcomes and shorter LOS.
5. Clinician's experience impacted outcomes. More experienced-- more efficient.
6. Outcomes do not predict Quality of Life or communication competence but they do predict patient satisfaction.
7. BOSS Outcomes could not be compared (benchmarked) to region or nation.
8. Advancing computer technology made data entry, integrated analyses , and large database possible but expensive. The lack of benchmarking without recurring investment and CMS recognition of ASHA NOMS dictated the transition to NOMS.
9. BOSS© outcomes were used: (a) to persuade payors to consider payments for Voice rehabilitation. (b) to demonstrate that clinical progress with Aphasic patients could not be accomplished without a minimal length of stay and treatment sessions. (c) to explain to the hospital administration the variance in clinical outcomes. (d) to demonstrate effectiveness of treatment options for Autism and Down's when costs and length of stay were difficult to manage. (e) to expand staff when clinical value (cost divided by GAIN) was good (f)

to meet JCAHO, CMS & BCBS standards of outcome reporting. (g) to argue the need to remove the CMS CAP on post-stroke rehabilitation. (h) to consider Cost-Effectiveness formulas for SLP treatment programs. (i) to facilitate an easy transition to ASHA NOM System

NATIONAL OUTCOME MEASUREMENT SYSTEM© 1997

In 1993 the American Speech-Language Hearing Association began a profession wide examination of treatment effectiveness in all healthcare environs.[9, 10] This was undertaken in response to its professional members, third party payors and their patients requests to have a broad based report card of the effectiveness and efficiency of our clinical services. In 1997 after several investigations and the efforts of a national task-force to establish a national data, the National Outcomes Measurement System (NOMS) of the American Speech-Language Hearing Association was developed. [6] The objective of the NOMS database was to demonstrate the "value of speech-language pathology services … provided to children and adults with communication and swallowing disorders" . [10]

The NOMS is based on a series of twenty one Functional Communication Measures that are organized as seven-point-equal-appearing interval clinical subjective scales. The seven point scales were standardized and developed with professional clinicians to clearly express the level of functional communication independence. Six of the communication performance scales are designed for childhood communication disorders and fifteen were developed for adults. Each scale delineates a communication function (i.e. articulation, comprehension, voice, pragmatics etc.) critical to identifying the severity of the disorders of communication. Level 1 on the functional communication scale (FCM) is the worst possible performance and level 7 is a normal functional level of communication performance. Each scale was carefully defined and revised to express the optimal agreement amongst professional clinicians as to the level of performance. (Appendix II)

Healthcare organizations with speech-language pathology service programs must register and train each of their clinicians to be certified to use the NOMS data collection system. The NOMS was designed to compare the clinical outcomes for a number of different communication disorders with a variety of demographic features (age, gender, medical disorder, length of stay, reimbursement, number of treatment, service delivery type etc.) . It is also designed to benchmark or compare treatment effectiveness or "value" of services provided between different facilities both regional and throughout the United States.

How are ASHA-NOMS© (est.1997) Different from the BOSS © Outcomes (est.1995)

a. NOMS measures the per cent of patients that make progress on the 7 point Functional Outcome Scales chosen for communication diagnosis.
b. BOSS measured the amount of progress that patients made on a 7 point outcome scales chosen for that specific communication diagnosis.
c. NOMS measures the percent of patients that did not make any progress.
d. BOSS measured the number of outliers (patients) who scored well below average at a particular clinical site and for a specific the communication diagnosis.
e. NOMS benchmarks a facility's outcomes to the regional or national outcomes.
f. BOSS did not benchmark their outcomes.
g. NOMS uses standardized (21) Functional Communication Measures for all communication diagnoses.
h. BOSS used sixty seven point scales developed by experienced clinicians specifically related to each communication diagnosis.
i. NOMS & BOSS both use length of stay, number of treatments, and admission scores to be compared with patient discharge scale scores.

The NOMS values the highly developed Functional Communication Measure as its key to estimating patient progress and clinical effectiveness. It's capacity to benchmark these outcomes to other facilities throughout the nation is unique and clearly advantageous. The NOMS is clearly the most reliable outcome measure and the gold standard in speech-language pathology clinical outcomes.

We learned a great deal from developing and using the BOSS outcome system as it prepared us to immediately adopt the NOMS system as our healthcare outcome system.

WHAT WE ARE LEARNING FROM ASHA- NOMS© AT BEAUMONT

Benchmarking Outcomes

We have been collecting NOMS outcome data for approximately seven years and have become accustomed to examining our outcomes compared to other clinical facilities in the Michigan region and the United States. Although we have only been collecting 3 to 6 year old children's outcomes for the past seven years, we are pleased to see that our clinical services produce as much if not more progress in our patients than the nation. The American Speech-Language Hearing Association, that operates the National Outcomes System (NOMS), provides these comparisons for any period of time that we may choose.

Table 4. NOMS© for Pre-Kindergarten at Beaumont, 2007-2013, N: 382

Pre-K Children 2007-2014	Beaumont	Nation
Articulation/Intelligibility	*86%	76%
Cognitive Orientation	87%	63%
Pragmatics	79%	62%
Spoken Language Comprehension	81%	67%
Spoken Language Production	83%	68%
Grand Average	82%	66%

**Percent of Patients Who Make Progress*

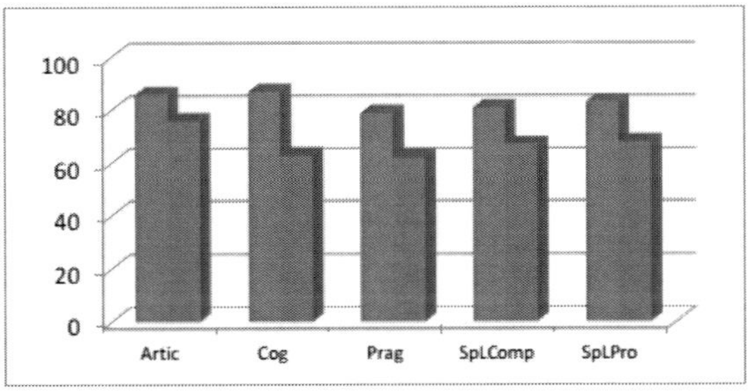

Bar Graph Illustration of Table 4

Benchmarked to the Nation N: 6138. Page 11.

In Table 4 we display all of our childhood patient (N:382) outcomes from 2007 through 2013 on four different functional communication measures (i.e. FCM: Articulation/Intelligibility, Cognitive Orientation, Pragmatics ,Spoken Language Comprehension and Spoken-Language Production) compared to the national benchmark (N: 6138). In all these FCM's we were able to exceed the average percent of patients making progress compared to the benchmark. We can average all these FCM's and report to our hospital administration that we average 82% for children making progress in our clinical services compared to the nation's 66%. The bar graph below Table 4 easily demonstrates these benchmarked comparisons. While it is comforting to report these clinical outcomes to our hospital and the public , these outcomes can certainly vary by a number of variables including case mix (i.e. different childhood diagnoses) admission severity and time in-treatment (90 days, 6 months or annually). Now that we have collected these large childhood populations rated on the NOMS (i.e. Beaumont N: 382 versus Nation N; 6138, accumulated during a seven year period 2007-2013) we can compare them to six month and twelve month outcomes and begin to consider the possible influences that affect these outcomes.

Table 5 demonstrates the adult outpatient outcomes in this same seven year period for four different Functional Communication Measures (FCM) also benchmarked against the nation , as reported by the American Speech-Language-Hearing Association. We exceed the percent of patients making progress in all four FCM's compared to the nation, but we are within the 95% confidence interval in Motor Speech, suggesting that our 76% and the nation's 73% are comparable or not significantly different. The nation's NOMS scores represent 23,437 patients across all the national facilities using NOMS and our patient population for this interval (2007-2013) is 517. These large differences can create percent progress variations. The ASHA NOMS provides patient demographics and case mix characteristics for the period samples requested. It is important to note that in these two populations, Beaumont's number of cerebrovascular disease patients were 46.6% of our caseload and only 17% of the nation's caseload. Further, our head injury population represented 26.1% of our caseload and only 3.7% of the nation's. Consequently 71% of our patients exhibited Aphasia and 16% presented with Dysarthria, compared to the nation's 11.4% of Aphasia diagnoses and 8.6% of Dysarthria diagnoses. The nation, during this period of time (2007-2013) reported that 59.9% of their adult caseload were treated for Dysphagia and only 9.8% of our patients were treated for Dysphagia. These variations in patient population mix will influence the overall Functional Communication Measures of patient progress.

Table 5. NOMS© for Adult Outpatients at Beaumont, 2007-2013, N: 517

Outpatient Adult 2007-2014	Beaumont	Nation
Spoken Language Comprehension	*82%	66%
Spoken Language Expression	82%	67%
Motor Speech	76%	73%
Memory	83%	65%
Grand Average	82%	69%

*Percent of Patients Who Make Progress

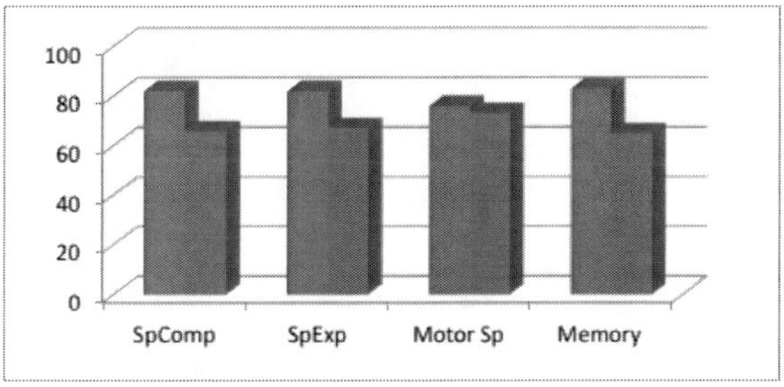

Bar Graph Illustration of Table 5

Benchmarked to the Nation N: 23,437. Page 11.

LEVELS OF PROGRESS ON THE NOMS©

Another way of possibly examining a facility's clinical effectiveness is to look at the number of patients who are not making any progress. In Chart #3 we illustrate our children's progress over this 2007-2013 period of time on one FCM (articulation/intelligibility). Compared to the nation, Beaumont demonstrated a smaller percent of patients making no progress, 13.9% than the nation 24.1%. Further we had a smaller percent of children making one level of progress (28.9%) compared to the nation (38.5%), however we made up for this reduction by demonstrating a larger percent of patients making multiple levels of progress (57.3%) compared to the nation at 37.4%. Our overall percent of children making progress for this FCM was 86.1% compared to the nation's 75.9%. These differences can usually be accounted for by differences in communication disorder diagnosis. Autism Spectrum Disorders and Down syndrome patients will make progress but are unlikely to make multiple levels of progress compared to Articulation and Language disorders.

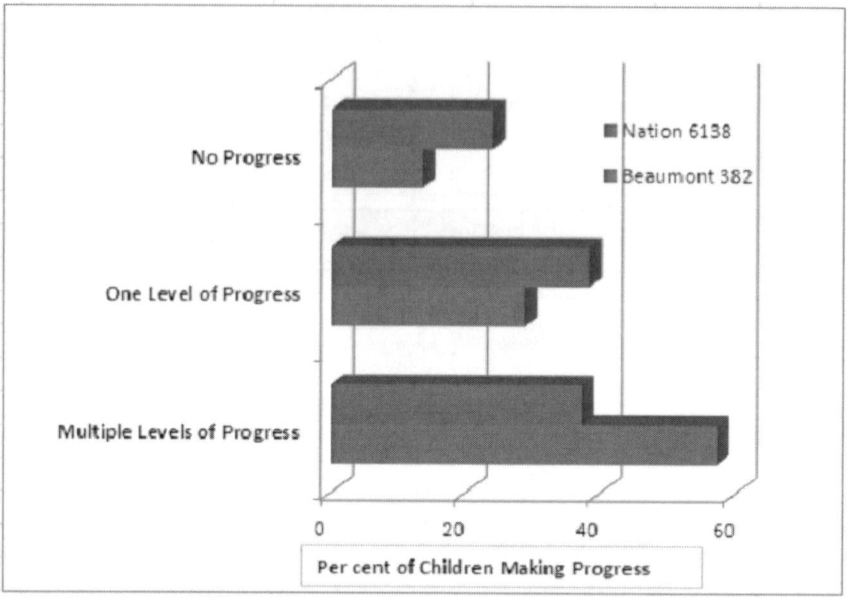

Per Cent of Children Making Progress Benchmarked to the Nation Page 12.

Chart 3. NOMS© Pre-Kindergarten at Beaumont, 2007-2013. Functional Communication Measure-Articulation/Intelligibility.

Population Demographics that Cause Variations in NOMS© Outcomes

In Table 6 we can clearly see how patient demographic characteristics can alter the potential NOMS score of "Per Cent of Patients that Make Progress". Here we compare a large patient population in our Adult Outpatient Clinics from 2007-2013 (N: 517) to the nation's patient population (N: 23,537). It is very clear that we see a different case-mix of adults who we treat compared to the nation. While our patient's average age range (60-69) is grossly comparable to the nation (i.e. 21% Beaumont and 16% Nation), our medical diagnoses and communication diagnoses are not similar (i.e. Beaumont at 46.5% CVA and 71% Aphasia, compared to 17.3% CVA and 11.4% Aphasia for the Nation). Further, a significantly larger number of our patients (97.3%)

are treated in a 46-90 minute treatment session compared to the Nation (19.6%). We might also have made greater progress with our patients because we treated them on average for a 57 day length of stay and the nation shows only 31 days of treatment. Finally, a large percentage of our patients are discharged directly to home (91.2%) compared to the nation at 38.4%, indicating that our patients did not have to return to the hospital, convalescent facility or skilled nursing facility. Our patients likely had fewer comorbidities and less severe disease and consequently less impairment or disability.

Table 6. NOMS© Demographic Characteristics of Adult Outpatients, 2007-2013 N: 517

Demographic Characteristic	Beaumont Health System	Nation
Age 60-69	21.2%	16.2%
Medical Diagnosis: Cerebrovascular Accident	46.5%	17.3%
Speech–Language Pathology Diagnosis:Aphasia	71%	11.4%
Per Cent of Patients Treatment Goals Met	61.5%	50.6%
Average Number of SLP Treatment Sessions	19.4	13.2
Length of SLP Treatment Session:46-90 minutes	97.3%	19.6%
Average Length of Stay	53.7	31.3
Discharge Disposition: Home	91.2%	38.4%

Benchmarked to the Nation, N: 23,537 Page 12.

BENCHMARKING BY REGION AND NATION

Another positive feature of the ASHA-NOMS is its capacity to compare our facility outcomes with the local region as well as the nation. These are very helpful comparisons for hospital administrators who are conscious of competition, and our third party payors who may be interested in relative clinical effectiveness and value. Table 7 briefly demonstrates our per cent of progress outcomes when compared to our Beaumont region (i.e. Michigan, Ohio, Illinois, Indiana and Pennsylvania). The Table demonstrates our Pre-Kindergarten population for the year 2010 on three FCM's (i.e. Articulation/intelligibility. Speech-Language Production, Speech-Language Comprehension). The numbers of patients in each FCM is relatively low as we discharged fewer children in this time period (2010) than usual. It is important to realize that some children are scored on one FCM or multiple FCM's depending on possible comorbidities or their specific communication disorder and the resulting treatment strategy.

Table 7. NOMS© Reporting Beaumont Outcomes for Pre-Kindergarten 2010

Functional Communication Measure	N	Beaumont % Patients/Progress	Region* % Patients/Progress	Nation % Patients/Progress
Articulation/Intelligibility	54	83 %	75%	75%
Speech-Lang/Production	50	92%	83%	70%
Speech-Lang/Comprehension	35	91%	84%	69%

3 Functional Communication Measures Benchmarked to Region and Nation Page 13.

The table demonstrates that we have greater numbers of children making progress compared to the Region and the Nation. For the Articulation/Intelligibility FCM we reported 83% of our children making progress and the Region and Nation tied at 75%. For the Speech-Language Production FCM Beaumont exhibited 92% of our children demonstrating progress with 83% for our Region and considerably less for the Nation at 70%. Again, these variations can be accounted for by patient population differences. One of the problems with using FCM's as the main feature of comparison in clinical treatment progress is that it covers a large potential variation in communication diagnoses.

IMPACT OF THE NUMBER OF TREATMENT SESSIONS ON NOMS© OUTCOMES

There is little disagreement among most clinicians that the more treatment sessions provided and/or allowed for by third party payors will affect the clinical outcomes. Chart 4 examines this premise in our Beaumont Pre-Kindergarten population (N: 382) compared to the Nation (N: 6138). The Chart illustrates that per cent of progress made by Beaumont and the Nation (Green and Red bars) increases with the greater number of treatment sessions provided.

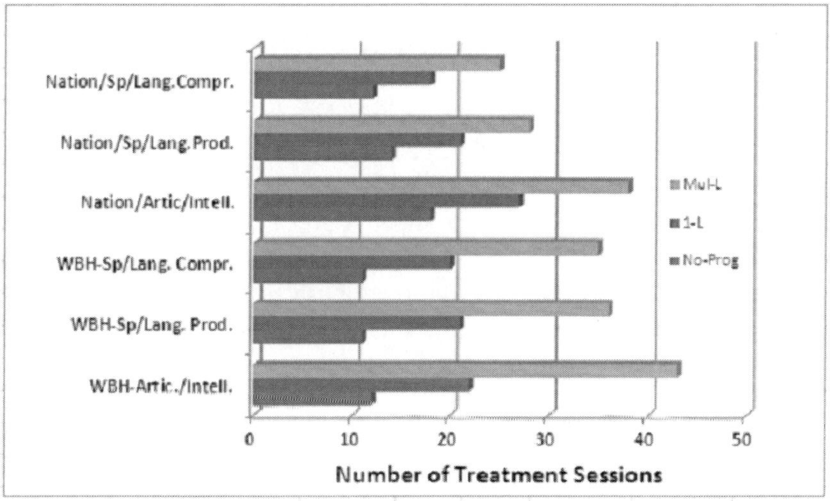

Treatment Sessions by Levels of Progress in Pre-K Children

	No-Prog	1-L	Mul-L
WBH-Artic./Intell.	12	22	43
WBH-Sp/Lang. Prod.	11	21	36
WBH-Sp/Lang. Compr.	11	20	35
Nation/Artic/Intell.	18	27	38
Nation/Sp/Lang.Prod.	14	21	28
Nation/Sp/Lang.Compr.	12	18	25

Table figures for Chart # 4

Comparing Progress by the Number of Treatment Sessions Beaumont , N:382. Benchmarked to the Nation N: 6138 Page 13.

Chart 4. NOMS© Pre-Kindergarten 4 Functional Communication Measures , 2007-2013.

The "no –progress" (blue bar) for all FCM's at Beaumont and the Nation also demonstrates that fewer treatment sessions were provided. The green bars or the multiple levels of progress designation clearly is correlated to the greater number of treatment sessions reported. These types of reports are extremely important in demonstrating to physicians, administrators, payors and politicians that cutting back the number of treatment sessions by staff reductions, failure to approve continuing treatment or reimbursement clearly reduces the demonstrated potential outcome gain.

Common Clinical Issues Defended by Outcomes

I. Dysphagia Outcomes Differ at Two Different Clinical Settings

We discovered several years ago that our swallowing rehabilitation programs at our main hospital (1070 beds) and our satellite hospital (418 beds) had noticeably different clinical outcomes. Analysis of our collected outcome data allowed us to observe that our larger, Level One Trauma hospital saw their swallowing patients within 8-10 hours of referral and began treatment immediately to prevent aspiration and to establish safe swallowing protocols. They also continued swallowing treatment after transfer to the acute inpatient rehabilitation unit.

The smaller community hospital clinicians saw their dysphagia patients 1-2 days after referral with less measured severity, in some cases, due to apparent spontaneous improvement. The staff was able to provide safe swallowing and diet recommendations and were able to discharge them without as much intervention. The outcomes revealed that patients seen earlier after referral were given more treatment due to a more severe admission level. These outcome findings suggest that each clinical environment has its own special patient care protocols depending on specific patient needs.

II. Therapy CAPS for Aphasic Patients

As has been stated earlier in this chapter, our outcome data, as well as a number of studies demonstrates that fewer treatment sessions with patients experiencing aphasia, produces lower discharge outcomes.[4, 5] Our outcome data suggests that a treatment program with 25-30 treatment sessions for speech and language pathology produces important gains in functional communication ability. Certainly, after 30 treatment sessions the outcome gain slows but is functionally significant.

Recently, Medicare caps, limitations on treatment, for aphasic patients have been implemented nationwide. It is our opinion that, NOMS clinical outcome data, when used to analyze improvement for this and other populations of neurologically impaired patients, clearly demonstrates that these caps significantly diminish the potential for recovery or critical functional speech and language skills. It should be noted that CMS recognizes NOMS as an approved outcome measurement system. [7].

III. Third Party Voice Treatment Guidelines

Payors have asked us if we could demonstrate, with our population of voice-impaired patients, the optimal number of treatment sessions to produce maximum gain or benefit to the patient. Apparently there were providers who seemed to bill for an unusually high number of treatment sessions for certain diagnoses. We were able to submit NOMS and BOSS outcome data that included mean length of stay and mean number of treatments, for a number of different vocal pathology diagnoses for a number of outpatient adults. This data has been very helpful in obtaining treatment pre-authorization for patients in need of vocal rehabilitation.

IV. Employer Monitoring of Quality Measures in Health Care

All hospital settings monitor quality of care. Our facility has asked all the clinical service departments to present evidence of clinical quality metrics and we have used our clinical outcomes in this regard for the past twenty years. For some departments this has meant costly acquisition of outcome measurement systems. We developed the BOSS© system in 1995 and then transitioned to the ASHA NOMS© in 2006 at virtually no cost to our department. Our hospital administration has readily accepted our NOMS outcome system and we often use these data to make the case for expanded resources. Our hospital system has asked us to simplify our outcomes reporting system and with the NOMS we can produce "grand average" dashboards or report cards that easily give us the ability to demonstrate and explain variations.

V. Answers Patient Questions on Clinical Prognosis

What clinician can say that they have never been asked the following questions by a patient:

How long will this treatment program take?
How many visits will be needed?
How much will this cost me or my payor?
Can I recover my normal functional voice, speech or language?
What increases my likelihood of a good clinical result?

Since we have used the BOSS© (1995) and the NOMS© (2006) we have been able , in certain clinical environments, to turn to our computers in the clinic and answer these questions. For example, we can tell a patient: from our outcome analyses in the past five years, that a person with vocal cord nodules has, on average, received 5-6 individual treatment sessions over a period 90 days and obtained a specific clinical improvement level. That usually mans on a scale of 7 being normal, the patient is likely to achieve a 5, or better in this time frame. We can also tell them that sometimes age, medical comorbidities and initial severity may influence this outcome. This has been a valuable clinical feature that can foster confidence and motivation in our patients.

Conclusion

Life is like riding a bicycle.
To keep your balance you must keep moving.
Albert Einstein, in a letter to his son Eduard, February 5, 1930 [11]

Clinical outcomes can be extremely important to clinical programs when building the case for measuring the value of speech and language rehabilitation [4, 5, 6, 2]. Outcome data collection can be used to demonstrate the critical benefits of our services to physicians, third party payors, administrators, government health care planners and our patients. [12] We can use outcome data to analyze and justify clinical programs by comparing effectiveness, efficiency and overall value. This information will be important as speech and language pathology is integrated into both national health planning initiatives and local accountable care organizations.

Clinical outcomes are not interpreted on "face value". They must be reported carefully with appropriate benchmarking and in sufficient numbers (reliability and correlation power) to be persuasive. They will be more effective when reported overtime, not in "brief periods" with no comparisons.

Clinical outcomes are powerful tools if carefully used. [4, 5, 9] They can be misinterpreted and rejected if not carefully presently and justified. The Beaumont Outcome Software System© (1995) was an early computer software program which attempted to account for treatment effectiveness over a ten year period of time in a large hospital based program. We learned some important lessons using the BOSS© and honed our skills at collecting and interpreting clinical outcomes. However, we were unable to benchmark our outcomes with local, regional or national programs. Further, we could not maintain the large and growing database in our hospital medical records system. The American Speech-Language Hearing Association's development and maintenance of their National Outcome Measurement System was an excellent service to the profession. Reporting clinical outcomes does not replace our extensive and growing professional armamentarium of standardized tests and assessments for a large variety of communicative diagnoses. [1, 2] In the future, the inevitable expansion of software and computer technology will allow us to develop even more analyses of patient performance, demographics and progress. Our profession must remain aware of these developments and make every attempt to harness these opportunities for the long-term benefits of our patients [2, 10].

References

[1] Shipley, KG, McAfee, J. Assessment in Speech-Language Pathology; A Resource Manual, 4ed. 2009, Delmar Cengage Learning, NY.

[2] Niewczyk P, Granger C, Brownscheidle, CN. The uniform data system for medical rehabilitation (UDSMR) and functional health assessment. *J. Med. Pers.* 10: 2012, 21-24.

[3] Lowit A, Kent RD . Assessment of Motor Speech Disorders. 1 edition. Plural Publishing Inc. October 2010 San Diego, Ca..

[4] Frattali, C. Editor, Measuring Outcomes in Speech-Language Pathology. Thieme Medical Publishers, New York, N.Y. 1998.

[5] Golper, LC, Frattali CM. Outcomes in Speech-Language Pathology, 2nd edition. Thieme Medical Publishers, New York, NY, 2013.

[6] Mullen, R. Evidence for Whom? ASHA's National Outcome Measurement System. *Journal of Communication Disorders* (37) 2004, 413-417.

[7] Frymark, T. NOMS Approved as Quality Measure Registry. American Speech-Language Hearing Association's National Center for Evidenced–Based Practice in Communication Disorders. *The ASHA Leader,* May 18, 2010.

[8] Merson R, Rolnick M, Weiner F. Beaumont Outcome Software System©. Parrot Software Inc. West Bloomfield, Michigan, 1995.

[9] Mullen, R, Schooling, T. The National Outcomes Measurement System for Pediatric Speech-Language Pathology. *Language, Speech, and Hearing Services in Schools,* January 2010, (41) 44-60.

[10] National Outcomes Measurement System, American Speech-Language Hearing Association, 1997-2012,.Robert Mullen, Dir., National Center for Evidence Based Practice in Communication Disorders, Rockville, Maryland. www.asha.org/nctecd/treatment_outcomes.htm

[11] Isaacson, W. EINSTEIN. Quote by Albert Einstein found on cover page. Simon & Schuster, New York, NY, 2007.

[12] Merson, RM, Rolnick MI. Cost-Effectiveness Analysis in Speech-Language Pathology Outcomes. Chapter 9 in Outcomes in Speech-Language Pathology, 2 ed. Thieme Medical Publishers, New York, NY, Pp. 2013, 183-201.

In: Speech, Language and Voice Pathology ISBN: 978-1-63321-958-8
Editor: Pablo Antonio Ysunza

Chapter 7

VELOPHARYNGEAL FUNCTION AND SPEECH. ANALYSIS OF SURGICAL OUTCOME IN YOUNG ADULTS WITH REPAIRED CLEFT PALATE AND RESIDUAL VELOPHARYNGEAL INSUFFICIENCY

Mirta Palomares*[*], *Drina Alvarez, Carlos Giugliano and Carolina Villena
Fundacion Dr. Alfredo Gantz, Santiago, Chile

ABSTRACT

The protocol for the evaluation and treatment of young adults with cleft palate at a Cleft Palate Center in Santiago, Chile is described. All the patients studied with this protocol were young adults present with residual velopharyngeal insufficiency (VPI) after palatal repair. All patients underwent a complete speech evaluation. Surgery for correcting VPI was planned individually in each case according to findings of videonasopharyngoscopy (VNP). All cases were operated on with a superiorly based pharyngeal flap. The surgical procedures were performed by the same surgeon in all cases.

Surgical outcomes of velopharyngeal function (VPF) were analyzed with postoperative VNP and a speech evaluation.

[*] Contact: mpaloma4@hotmail.com

Patients with normal articulation before surgery showed adequate VPF one month after the pharyngeal flap was performed. None of these cases required Speech & Language Pathology (SLP) treatment.

None of the patients with compensatory articulation disorder (CAD) preoperatively showed adequate VPF one month after the pharyngeal flap operation. All these cases required SLP treatment including biofeedback with VNP. After a six-month period of SLP treatment and biofeedback, sixty – three percent of these patients achieved similar results as the group of patients with normal articulation before surgery. After a follow-up period of 6 months, a total of 79% of the cases showed satisfactory results of VPF during speech. Most patients showed good compliance and motivation for treatment.

Keywords: Cleft palate, Speech, Surgery

INTRODUCTION

Velopharyngeal Insufficiency (VPI) refers to any structural alteration of the soft palate and the pharyngeal walls where there is not enough tissue for a complete closure of the velopharyngeal sphincter (VPS) during the production of oral phonemes [1]. The percentage of patients with residual VPI following cleft palate (CP) repair varies from center to center, but in general it is estimated that 10 - 20% of patients with cleft palate will present with VPI post palatal repair. [2-4]

The presence of residual VPI affects various parameters of speech and voice resonance. The characteristic symptomatology is the presence of obligatory errors including: hypernasality, nasal emission, weak oral consonants and compensatory articulation disorder (CAD). [5]

Several surgical techniques for correcting VPI have been described. The selection of a specific technique for each patient depends on closure pattern as observed by videonasopharyngoscopy (VNP) and videofluoroscopy (VF). The most commonly used surgical techniques for correcting VPI include: Modified Orticochea's pharyngoplasty or lateral flaps operation; surgical increase of the posterior pharyngeal wall; superiorly based pharyngeal flap; and secondary surgical repair of velar muscles. [6]

It has been reported that surgery for correcting VPI yields better outcomes when it is performed at an early age, ideally before entering the preschool system, when communication demands increase. At this stage, around 4 years of age, children have usually acquired a greater number of phonemes and show better compliance for performing procedures which allow a full assessment of VPF including an instrumental evaluation of the VPS through VNP and VF. It has been reported that when VPI is corrected early, there is an improvement in over 90% of the cases. [7]

CAD refers to speech errors derived from unconscious patient attempts to produce a phoneme, usually a high intraoral pressure consonant sound. In these cases, articulation placement is displaced closer to the sound source, usually to the pharynx or the glottis. The most common compensatory errors are: the glottal stop and the pharyngeal fricative. [1] CAD is present more frequently in patients with severe VPI [8]. CAD significantly affects intelligibility.

In cases of CAD, prognosis is less favorable since speech sound errors are incorporated into Linguistic rules. Thus, it becomes much more difficult to change brain motor engrams, affecting surgical outcome and extending the total time of Speech & Language Pathology (SLP) intervention [1]. It has been described that articulatory placement and manner are more malleable at earlier ages. Therefore, even in cases of CAD, surgical correction of VPI can decrease total time of SLP treatment. Also, correcting hypernasality can provide more confidence for developing speech skills and abilities. [9, 10]

Currently, there are health programs and international organizations that promote and support early and timely care of patients with cleft palate (CP). Centers with more experience and better results usually perform the primary surgeries of lip and palate before one year of age. Early repair of the palate is recommended in order to minimize speech disorders. [11] Unfortunately there are patients that for various reasons do not have access to multidisciplinary treatment, thus hampering rehabilitation and integration into society.

Young adults with CP usually have an increased frequency of social, occupational and emotional limitations. [12] These limitations negatively affect the rehabilitation process. In these cases, CAD, VPI, palatal fistulae, abnormal dental occlusion and septal deviation are common findings. All these factors significantly affect quality of life [13, 14].

Some reports studying adult patients describe that there are no significant changes in the speech intelligibility following VPI surgery. This finding seems to be related with the articulatory errors that directly affect VPS motion during speech. Even with an appropriately planned surgical treatment, hypernasality is corrected in only 75% of the cases. [8]

Hamlen (1970) pointed out that poor surgical result in adults can be associated with greater difficulty for acquiring and using new speech abilities, as well as lack of family support. [15]

Several strategies can be used for the management of CAD including: Phonological approach; auditory biofeedback; and biofeedback with VNP. Traditionally it has been described that most patients with CAD respond positively to conventional speech intervention. Witzel et al, (1989) demonstrated that patients with velopharyngeal dysfunction associated with CAD undergoing pharyngeal flap, achieved a consistent closure of the VPS in connected speech after biofeedback therapy using VNP. [16]

Endoscopic feedback would be indicated for patients who do not respond to conventional intervention or those who are progressing too slowly. Fast and consistent positive results have been reported in patients with CAD who have undergone endoscopic biofeedback. With the use of this technique, CAD can be corrected in a few sessions. It has been reported that endoscopic biofeedback therapy seems to be superior to conventional intervention for treating velopharyngeal dysfunction associated with CAD. [17]

Direct visualization of the VPS supports articulation therapy creating a greater impact on the patient, improving learning and reducing total time of therapy. [16, 18]

Young adults with residual VPI require an interdisciplinary management which basically considers the same procedures for evaluation and treatment as used in children, but with some modifications in its application, considering anatomical and emotional differences, as well as self - motivation.

The purpose of this chapter is to describe a protocol for treating VPI in young adults, considering individualized surgical planning and SLP intervention.

Materials and Methods

Patients

Patients were recruited at the Fundacion Dr. Alfredo Gantz in Santiago, Chile, from 2005 to 2013. All cases who met the following inclusion criteria were included in the study group: patients with cleft lip and CP or isolated CP; older than 17 years; without associated syndromes; with normal hearing; present with residual VPI after initial palatal repair; without fistulae; without further surgical procedures for correcting VPI other than the initial palatal repair.

All cases were assessed by the cleft palate team. They were guided by personal motivation and they committed themselves to undergo all necessary evaluations and interventions.

Speech Assessment

Each patient was evaluated before and after the surgery by the same Speech & Language Pathologist at the Fundación Gantz. The professional conducting the evaluations had more than 10 years of clinical experience in the evaluation and treatment of patients with craniofacial anomalies.

Severity of the VPI, presence of CAD and size of the gap as observed by VNP before the surgical procedure were assessed.

It should be pointed out that before performing the VNP, all patients should be able to produce at least 2 high oral pressure consonant phonemes with adequate placement during the repetition of syllables and isolated words. Therefore, SLP treatment was provided before the procedure whenever it was considered necessary to do so.

The VPI was classified according to the severity of the hypernasality and nasal emissions (Table 1).

Table 1. Classification of VPI according to severity

VPI Severity	VPI Symptomatology
Without VPI	Normal Velopharyngeal Function; absence of hypernasality*; No nasal emission.
Mild VPI	Mild hypernasality - nasal turbulence.
Moderate VPI	Moderate Hypernasality – as perceived during the production of vowel sounds. Audible nasal emissions during production of most of the high pressure consonant phonemes.
Severe VPI	Severe hypernasality during the production of vowel sounds and oral consonant phonemes. Nasal emission in all high pressure consonant phonemes. Low pressure in oral consonant phonemes. Facial grimaces or movements associated with nasal emission.

* Severity of hypernasality was classified according to a previously reported 4-point scale [18].

Speech was classified according to the presence or absence of CAD. No CAD was considered as the condition in which the patient had normal articulation placement in all speech contexts, despite the presence of hypernasality; CAD was considered when articulation placement was abnormal in different contexts such as repetition of syllables, words, sentences and automatic or spontaneous speech.

Instrumental Evaluation of VPI

Pre and post-operative evaluation of the VPI was performed by VNP. A flexible scope with a diameter of 3.5mm at the tip was used. This procedure was carried out by the same Otolaryngologist and SLP in all cases. A standardized speech sample was used including isolated phonemes, connected speech, automatic speech and sustained fricative phoneme sounds [19]. All procedures were recorded for a thorough further analysis. Size and shape of the gap and velopharyngeal closure pattern during speech were assessed. Ten-percent gaps or bubbling without a discernable gap were considered as small gaps. Gaps larger than 10% but less than 40% were considered as medium size gaps. Gaps larger than 40% were considered as large gaps.

Surgical Procedure

Each surgical procedure for correcting VPI was planned individually according to findings of VNP. In order to prevent postoperative airway obstruction, other factors were also considered for designing the surgical plan, including adenoid and/or tonsil hypertrophy, and nasal septum deviation.

A superiorly base pharyngeal flap would be indicated in cases present with circular or sagittal patterns. The width of the flap was designed to match the maximum displacement of the lateral pharyngeal walls during the production of the speech sample.

A lateral flaps pharyngoplasty would be indicated in cases with a predominantly coronal shape of the gap. Posterior Pharyngeal wall increase using cartilage or fat was used in cases with coronal or circular gaps not greater than 10%.

Post-surgical complications were assessed in all cases.

Speech Therapy Post-Surgery

Postoperative SLP treatment was implemented according with the SLP evaluation which was routinely performed one month after surgery in all cases. Patients with satisfactory outcome of speech and VPF did not receive further treatment. However, they were followed up monthly for a period of 6 months. Patients with postoperative unsatisfactory outcomes as determined by presence of CAD and/or present with incomplete velopharyngeal closure during speech received SLP treatment including 2 modalities: Articulation placement intervention provided in a 45-minutes session once-per-week and a separate biofeedback 30-minutes session also once-per-week.

The intervention addressing articulation placement and manner was aimed to correct abnormal articulation patterns and carry over adequate articulation into connected speech. Initially, imitations and repetitions strategies were used. Further on, generalization strategies were used in order to enhance carrying over into connected speech. These strategies included reading aloud, singing, conversational speech, and role – play. [16]

Biofeedback therapy included recognition and identification of velopharyngeal structures on the VNP image; analysis of VPS motion during swallowing, blowing and speech; and finally, analysis of VPS motion during the production of oral consonant phonemes with best and worst velopharyngeal closure. Also, during the biofeedback sessions, some of the strategies used during the articulation intervention were also incorporated as velopharyngeal motion was being observed on the screen.

Discharge

The criteria for definite discharge were: normal articulation placement and manner during conversational speech and normal VPF in different speech contexts.

Ethical Aspects

This study was approved by the Ethics Committee of Fundación Gantz. All patients were recruited in this Center. The study was conducted in accordance with the ethical standards of the 1964 Helsinki Declaration. Each patient was carefully briefed about the diagnostic procedures, the surgical procedure that would be performed and the eventual subsequent SLP treatment that would be provided. All patients signed an informed consent before being accepted as participants.

RESULTS

Fourteen surgical procedures were performed. All patients were older than 17 years of age. Seven patients were males and 7 patients were females. Age range was 17 – 35 years of age. Mean age was 24 years of age. No intraoperative or immediate postoperative complications were detected.

All cases studied for this protocol presented with a circular pattern. Thus, all cases were operated on with a superiorly based pharyngeal flap. No other surgical procedure was performed in this series. Three patients were operated on with a narrow flap; six patients were operated on with a medium flap; and 5 patients required a wide flap. The width of the flap was designed to match maximum lateral pharyngeal wall displacement during speech as observed by VNP. (See Table 2).

Forty-three percent of the patients studied for this protocol did not show CAD preoperatively. All these cases demonstrated adequate VPF as determined by the SLP assessment one month postoperatively. All these cases did not require any further treatment and were discharged.

The remaining 57% of the cases demonstrated CAD preoperatively. None of these cases were able to achieve adequate VPF one month postoperatively (See Table 2). All these patients underwent further postoperative SLP treatment and biofeedback with VNP. Five out of these 8 cases achieved adequate articulation and VPF after an intervention period of 6 months. Finally, the remaining 3 cases which persisted with inadequate VPF and/or abnormal articulation placement showed mild or moderate hypernasality during spontaneous – connected speech. One of these cases demonstrated a flap with scar tissue which decreased the width of the flap. In this case, by using "forced" articulation placement during the production of isolated words, both ports of the flap looked practically occluded as observed by VNP. However, during spontaneous – connected speech, both lateral pharyngeal walls failed to make tight contact with the lateral – free borders of the flap causing hypernasality and inconsistent nasal emission. Another patient presented with a very narrow flap which could not achieve complete closure not even during the production of isolated words. This case required a new surgical procedure.

Table 2. Patient's characteristics and results of the pre and postoperative evaluations

Patients	Age (years)	Cleft Type	Presence of CAD	Preoperative VPI Severity	Preoperative size of the gap (%)	Selected flap witdth	Postoperative VPI (1 months)	VPI severity after SLP treatment (6 months)	Discharged
1	22	UCLP	Yes	Moderate	20	Medium	Moderate	Without VPI	Yes
2	20	CCP	No	Mild	10	Narrow	Without VPI	-	Yes
3	17	ICP	Yes	Severe	50	Width	Moderate	Without VPI	Yes
4	17	ICP	No	Moderate	30	Medium	Without VPI	-	Yes
5	34	BCLP	Yes	Severe	80	Width	Severe	Mild	No
6	18	UCLP	Yes	Severe	70	Width	Severe	Mild to moderate	No
7	24	BCLP	No	Mild	10	Narrow	Without VPI	-	Yes
8	35	UCLP	Yes	Moderate	40	Medium	Severe	Mild	No
9	23	UCLP	No	Mild	10	Narrow	Without VPI	-	Yes
10	20	CCP	No	Moderate	30	Medium	Without VPI	-	Yes
11	32	CCP	Yes	Moderate	40	Medium	Mild	Without VPI	Yes
12	20	BCLP	No	Moderate	20	Medium	Without VPI	-	Yes
13	26	BCLP	Yes	Severe	80	Width	Severe	Without VPI	Yes
14	23	UCLP	Yes	Severe	80	Width	Severe	Without VPI	Yes

Key: UCLP = unilateral cleft lip and palate, BCLP = bilateral cleft lip and palate, ICP = incomplete cleft palate, CCP = complete cleft palate.

Finally, the third patient presented with a flap with an apparent adequate width, good lateral walls motion but it was not possible to achieve a complete seal during connected speech after 6 months of SLP intervention and biofeedback sessions. This patient did not return for a follow up visit in which further surgical treatment would have been discussed. It should be emphasized that these 3 cases with postoperative residual hypernasality and nasal emission demonstrated CAD and a severe VPI preoperatively.

In the overall analysis of the group of patients studied for this chapter, seventy-nine-percent (11 of 14) of the cases achieved a satisfactory outcome following the pharyngeal flap operation and a period not longer than 6 months of postoperative SLP treatment including biofeedback sessions with VNP.

Conclusion

The purpose of this chapter was to assess speech and VPF outcome in young adults undergoing surgery aimed to correct VPI.

Poor results have been reported in adult patients who undergo pharyngeal flap surgery [11], hence leading some cleft palate teams to question the implementation of surgery for correcting VPI in this age group. However, a higher success rate (80 - 90%) was reported [20] when general population including children and adults were studied. Another report [8], describes that in young adults, an adequate surgical planning before performing a pharyngeal flap can increase the success rate up to 75%.

The results of this chapter show that 43% of young adults showed improvement of speech and VPF one month following pharyngeal flap surgery. All of these cases were from the Group of patients without CAD. This percentage rose to 79% after SLP intervention aimed to correct CAD including VNP biofeedback.

A relationship between CAD and lateral pharyngeal wall motion has been reported in several papers. [13-14, 16] This could explain why SLP treatment and endoscopic biofeedback increase velopharyngeal closure after a tailor made pharyngeal flap. Moreover, an aberrant lateral walls movements with outward displacement during the production of some fricative phonemes has been reported in cases of CAD [21]. Endoscopic biofeedback seems a safe a reliable tool for correcting this abnormal velopharyngeal motion during speech. In the group of patients studied for this chapter, patients without CAD demonstrated mild VPI with sizes of the gap equal or below 30%. (See Table 2).

It has been reported that endoscopic biofeedback can increase lateral walls motion [22]. Thus, the closure pattern can be modified from a circular pattern into a more sagittal pattern. In the patients studied for this chapter, 5 cases managed to successfully mobilize the lateral pharyngeal walls during speech, resulting in a significant improvement in their speech and VPF. As described by Witzel et al. (1989) [16] some patients have the potential to increase movement of the lateral pharyngeal walls with adequate training. However, it should be pointed out that some of our patients failed to achieve adequate lateral pharyngeal walls motion despite the use of endoscopic biofeedback. Moreover, some of our patients were able to increase motion during the production of isolated words but they were not able to consistently carry over this improvement into conversational speech.

Correction of CAD should consider the use of effective strategies of SLP intervention. In adult patients, the use of biofeedback therapy with VNP seems a valuable tool which can provide a direct visualization of the VPS during speech. Patients undergoing this procedure usually increase awareness of VPS motion which facilitates carrying over the improvement into conversational speech. Also, the integration of auditory and visual inputs effectively decreases total time of the SLP intervention. [23]. Nonetheless, it should be considered that endoscopic biofeedback is an additional tool which should be used as a complement to conventional strategies aimed to correct articulation placement.

When articulation strategies including endoscopic biofeedback are used for 6 months following pharyngeal flap surgery, patients with CAD can achieve similar final outcomes as those of patients who did not present CAD preoperatively.

Adult patients often present with various physical and/or functional alterations in addition to preferences and motivations that are usually related with social aspects and job issues. [12-14]Some patients prefer an intervention for improving communication skills, whereas others are more motivated to improve aesthetic appearance, and dental occlusion. It is important for the cleft palate team to consider the individual needs and points of view of each patient. In the group of patients studied for this chapter, all patients sought treatment by personal motivation and the most common goal was to improve communication.

From the results described in this chapter, it is evident that VPI in young adults should be addressed with a specifically designed treatment plan. Anatomy of the palate, degree of VPI, presence of CAD, size of the defect, and patient motivation should be carefully assessed in each case.

The implementation of the Protocol described herein can provide a better guide for diagnosis and treatment. Thus, an appropriate surgical and SLP intervention plan can be designed, improving final outcome.

From the analysis of the group of young adults studied for this chapter, it seems that those patients present with VPI and CAD who do not show an appropriate motivation for following the long term management program, cannot be considered good candidates for surgery.

Although the results described for the group of young adults analyzed for this chapter are promising, it will be necessary to study larger groups of patients with different characteristics in order to support the conclusions of this study. It should be emphasized that young adults with appropriate personal motivation for improvement have an acceptable chance for a favorable outcome. However, as mentioned herein, the best results seem to be associated with absence of CAD preoperatively, as well as the presence of small and medium sizes of gap at the VPS during speech.

REFERENCES

[1] Ysunza, A., Pamplona, M. (2002).Diagnóstico y Tratamiento de los trastornos de articulación en el niño con paladar hendido. México: Editorial Porrúa.

[2] Shprintzen, R. (1996).Cleft palate management: a multidisciplinary approach (Vol.5).St Luis, EEUU: Mosby Yearbook.

[3] Altmann, E. (1997). Fissuras Labiopalatinas. Sao Paulo: Pró-fono.

[4] Marrinan, E., LaBrie, R. & Mulliken, J. (1998). Velopharyngeal function in nonsyndromic cleft palate: relevance of surgical technique, age at repair, and cleft type. *Cleft Palate Journal*.21, 263-269.

[5] Golding- Kushner, K.J. (2001). Therapy Techniques for cleft palate Speech and related disorders. New Jersey: Singular Thomson Learning.

[6] Giugliano, C. (2008). Tratamiento de la IVF. En L. Monasterio, Tratamiento Interdisciplinario de las Fisuras Labio Palatinas.Santiago, Chile: Fundación Gantz, 407-418.

[7] Argamaso, R.V., Shprintzen, R.J., Strauch, B., Lewin, M.L., Daniller, A.I., Ship, A.G. & Croft, C.B. (1980). The role of lateral pharyngeal wall movement in pharyngeal flap surgery. *Plast. Reconstr. Surg*. 66, 214-219.

[8] Hall, C.D., Golding-Kushner, K.J., Argamaso, R. & Strauch, B. (1991). Pharyngeal Flap Surgery in Adults. *Cleft Palate J.* 28 (2), 179-183.

[9] Riski, J.E. (1979). Articulation skills and oral-nasal resonance in children with pharyngeal flaps. *Cleft Palate J.* 16, 421-428.

[10] Fletcher, S.G. (1978). Diagnosing speech disorders from cleft palate. New York: Grune & Stratton.

[11] Ortiz-Monasterio, F., Serrano, R., Barrera, G.P., Rodriguez-Hoffman, H. & Vinageras, E. (1966). A study of untreated adult cleft patients. *Plast. Reconstr. Surg*. 38, 37-41.

[12] Mani, M., Carlsson, M. & Marcusson, A.(2010). Quality of Life Varies with Gender and Age among Adults Treated for Unilateral cleft Lip and Palate. *Cleft Palate J.* 47 (5), 491- 498.

[13] Marcusson, A., Akerlind, I. & Paulin, G. (2001). Quality of Life in Adults with Repaired Complete Cleft Lip and Palate. *Cleft Palate J.* 38 (4).

[14] Bing, C., Searle, Y., Jeremy, A., Richard, B., Sharp, I.& Slater, R. (2008).The Continuing Multidisciplinary Needs of Adults Patients With Cleft Lip and/or Palate. *Cleft Palate Craniofac. J.* 45(6), 633-638.

[15] Hamlen, M. (1970). Speech changes after pharyngeal flap surgery. *Plast. Reconstr. Surg*. 46, 437-444.

[16] Witzel, M.A., Tobe, J. & Salyer, K.E. (1989). The use of videonasopharyngoscopy for biofeedback therapy in adults after pharyngeal flap surgery. *Cleft Palate J.* 26, 129-134.

[17] Brunner, M., Stellzig-Eisenhauer, A., Pröschel, U., Verres, R. & Komposch, G. (2005).The Effect of Nasopharyngoscopy Biofeedback in Patients With Cleft Palate and Velopharyngeal Dysfunction. *Cleft Palate Craniofac J.* 42(6), 649-57.

[18] Monasterio, L. (2008). Tratamiento Interdisciplinario de las Fisuras Labio Palatinas. Santiago, Chile: Fundación Gantz.

[19] Henningsson, G., Kuehn, D., Sell, D., Sweeney, T., Trost-Cardamone, J. Whitehill,T. (2008). Universal Parameters for Reporting Speech Outcomes in individuals with cleft Palate. *Cleft Palate Cran*. J.45 (1), 1-17.

[20] Patel, P., Mrasseschi, M. & McGraw, E. (2012). Surgical treatment of Velopharyngeal dysfunction. Retrieved June 6, 2014 from http://emedicine.medscape.com/article/873018-overview#showall.

[21] Pamplona, M.C., Ysunza, A., Silva, A. & Jiménez, G. (2000). Videonasofaringoscopía para retroalimentación del habla en pacientes con paladar hendido. *An. Otorrinolaringol.* Mex. 45(2), 46-50.

[22] Siegel-Sadewitz, VL, Shprintzen, RJ. (1982). Nasopharyngoscopy of the normal velopharyngeal sphincter: an experiment of biofeedback. *Cleft palate J.* 19: 194-200.
[23] Shprintzen, R.J. & Golding-Kushner, K. (1989). Advances in evaluating velopharyngeal insufficiency. *North Am. Clin.Otolaryngol.* 22, 519-536.

In: Speech, Language and Voice Pathology
Editor: Pablo Antonio Ysunza
ISBN: 978-1-63321-958-8

Chapter 8

STRATEGIES FOR TREATING PHONOLOGIC DISORDER IN CHILDREN WITH CLEFT PALATE

Maria C. Pamplona[1] and Santiago Morales[2]
[1]Hospital Gea González. Mexico City
[2]The Penn State University, PA, US

ABSTRACT

Children with cleft palate (CCP) may be at risk for articulation disorders. These articulation patterns are known as compensatory articulation disorder (CAD) and are generally regarded as compensatory behaviors secondary to velopharyngeal insufficiency (VPI).

Some authors consider these behaviors as a phonologic disorder.

Whole language principles consider that there is an interaction between the phonological rules and other language rule systems. An articulation problem is far more complex in nature than a phonetic analysis would suggest, and during intervention, phonologic information should not be separated from the other areas of language, such as pragmatics or syntax. Thus, within the same activity, several pieces of information about all areas of language, including phonologic information are provided.

Scaffolding strategies can be useful for correcting placement and manner of articulation. Sometimes, it is difficult to know which strategy would be best option for a specific moment. Few authors have specified the expected time to apply each strategy in order to improve effectiveness. However, when studying the efficacy of these strategies for treating CAD in CCP, some result more adequate depending on the specific stage of speech development or severity of articulation impairment.

In this chapter some scaffolding strategies for phonologic intervention will be described and some ideas for using them in communicative situations in relationship with higher organizational levels of language processing.

Keywords: Cleft palate; Speech; Language; Rehabilitation; Therapy

Introduction

Articulation disorders in children may be either phonetic or phonologic in nature. Phonetic disorders are related to inaccurate learning or anatomic, physiologic or/and motor deficits. In contrast, phonologic disorders are considered to be linguistically based and reflect difficulty in the child's organization and representation of the sound system of language. [1 – 3]

Children with cleft palate (CCP) may have an articulation disorder. Certain articulation disorders are generally regarded as compensatory behaviors secondary to velopharyngeal insufficiency (VPI). These errors include dysfunction not only of the velopharyngeal sphincter, but also of the entire vocal tract and higher levels of articulation control in the central nervous system. [4, 5] For example, plosive sounds such as /p/ or /k/ might be attempted by substituting a glottal stop. These abnormal articulation patterns are usually referred as compensatory articulation disorder (CAD). CAD severely affects intelligibility and usually requires a prolonged period of speech therapy. [6, 7]

Compensatory Articulation: Phonetic or Phonologic in Nature?

Several authors have described that cleft palate patients are at risk for phonetic based problems due to the structural deviations associated with clefting. [8, 9] However, cleft palate children may be also at risk for phonologic disorders. [10]

A phonetic disorder occurs when the movements of the articulators, such as the lips, tongue, palate, or resonating cavity are altered from a normal or typical production. A compensation such as glottal production or CAD would be considered phonetic, as the child with velopharyngeal insufficiency attempted to produce the sound in an alternative manner to compensate for the inability to establish intraoral air pressure because of the cleft. [10] Because the glottal production reflected an obvious and productive compensation, the problem was viewed as phonetic and articulation became the main topic in intervention. However, only a small or moderate percentage of children with repaired cleft palate exhibit CAD. Most patients, following the repair, produce the more typical pattern and no articulation delays or deviations are seen. [6]

The finding that a small percentage of patients continue to produce CAD despite the early and effective repair of the cleft suggests that some factor other than the inability to establish sufficient intraoral air pressure is contributing to the development and maintenance of this articulatory pattern. Most of the palatal repairs are completed between 12 and 18 months of age, or at the time when first words appear. The appearance of words suggests that by this age children are already establishing a phonological system, or a set of linguistic rules that map the phonetic patterns of speech to the sound and syllable patterns of meaningful language. Thus, what had been a compensatory strategy for approximating sounds heard in the environment during early stages of babbling for some patients becomes incorporated into the phonological rule system before the surgery is completed. Following surgery, when the child is quite capable of producing the plosive sounds or other speech patterns in a more typical manner, the child continues to produce the CAD form because it had become integrated with the language rules instead of the correct pattern. At this point, what began as a phonetic compensation had become a phonological rule. As a generative and productive rule, the articulatory production would not change until the rule is changed, despite the change in the physical capability to produce the sound correctly.

Evidence for the contention that many of the speech problems of cleft palate children are phonological rather than phonetic can be found in two studies. Chapman in 1993, compared articulation errors produced by children with cleft palate to age-matched and younger groups of typically developing children using a phonological analysis. A phonological analysis examines errors for patterns, such as deleting or modifying sound production patterns according to regularities or "rules." Her findings indicated that children with cleft palate produced the same types of phonological process errors as the younger typically developing children, but they maintained these process errors longer than the age-matched peers. She also found that the children with cleft palate used the phonological process of backing with greater frequency and for more sounds than did the typically developing children. She concluded that these findings suggested that the articulation errors of children with cleft palate were of the same phonological nature as the typically developing children, and that the high occurrence of backing indicated that compensatory gestures had become incorporated into the phonological rules of the subjects. [10]

In the second study, Pamplona et al, in 1999, treated children with CAD following surgery in either a phonetic or a phonological treatment approach. In the phonetic approach children were taught correct production of the error sounds through modeling and reinforcement, using a repetitive drill for a single phoneme until it was mastered. In the phonological condition, multiple errors were targeted simultaneously by focusing on a process, such as producing phonemes in a more frontal position. Thus, three phonemes that had been produced as a glottal stop, such as /k/, /t/, and /p/ were treated simultaneously as sounds requiring more frontal posturing. The phonemes were taught and practiced in a meaningful language context such as storybook reading. Results indicated that while both groups improved their speech, the phonological group achieved normal speech production on average one year sooner than did the phonemic group, which required 2 1/2 years of therapy. Addressing the phonological rules resulted in faster learning of the target productions and more rapid incorporation into the language rules and thus more immediate carryover into conversational speech. [6]

These findings suggest that many of the articulation problems in children with repaired cleft palate currently viewed as phonetic may actually be phonological as early as one year of age. It also implies that during speech assessment and intervention, some additional phonologic analysis and specific strategies should be employed.

Speech intervention in CCP with a phonetic approach considers articulation learning as a specific time of motor learning. Moreover, errors in articulation must be seen as disruptions at some level of the relatively peripheral articulatory processes. Consequently, some therapy procedures are based almost exclusively on the notion that articulation errors are due to faulty control of the articulators. [11, 2] In contrast, in a phonologic approach the children must learn more than just a set of complex articulatory patterns associated with words. They must learn a complete system of phonology. Furthermore, several authors have proposed that some central, cognitive-phonological processing must be included in any description of phonological acquisition. [1, 2]

WHOLE LANGUAGE MODEL. INTEGRATING PHONOLOGY IN A WHOLE

The phonological approach for treating compensatory articulation disorder in cleft palate patients does not necessarily rejects well-established principles underlying traditional approaches for articulation disorders. In contrast, articulation must be recognized as a critical aspect of speech sound development under any theory. Consequently, phonological principles should be considered as adding new dimensions and a new perspective to an old problem, not simply as refuting established principles. [2]

Because the phonological system is integrally integrated with the language system, and because faster progress was made when treatment for CAD was more successful when conducted in the meaningful language context of storybook reading, it is also suggested that the language of children with CAD should also be assessed. Hoffman, in 1992, stated that children's speech sound production and perception errors are related not only to phonological knowledge, but also to higher organizational levels of language processing. He also mentions some research findings indicating that children who have difficulty learning phonology also show similar difficulties for learning morphological, syntactic, and semantic regularities of language as well. Hoffman and his colleagues in a series of studies showed that children with phonological disorders made greater progress in both articulation and in language measures such compared to children in treatment approaches that focused on phonological patterns practiced outside of a meaningful language context. [3, 12]

Other researchers have identified language problems in children with cleft palate, including syntax (i.e., grammar), morphology, and vocabulary. [4, 13 – 15]

These findings suggest that many of the language problems actually exhibited by children with CAD may be overlooked when the speech disorder is viewed from a phonetic rather than a phonological perspective. In many cases, there is an interaction between the phonological rules and other language rule systems, so that an articulation problem is really far more complex in nature than a phonetic analysis would suggest.

Pamplona and Ysunza (2000) also found a relationship between CAD and the child´s language system, including the ability to use semantic, syntactic, and discourse elements of language rules to express meaning. In this study, they found that children with CAD differ in their overall development of language, and not just speech productions, from children with repaired cleft palates that do not showed the CAD speech patterns. These findings suggest that it would be reasonable to provide children with CAD with a more global treatment including linguistic aspects. Treating only the articulation disorders does not seem enough for these patients. It seems more appropriate to consider higher levels of language including abstract thought and reading and writing activities. [16]

For understanding the interaction between CAD and higher levels of language organization we have to consider that children learn language in the context of events such as eating or bathing routines. [12] As they learn the rules, actions and objects are associated with the events, they map words to the visual event. These words would include many levels and descriptions of the ongoing actions and related objects.

Once the words are integrated with the event, they serve to add complexity and abstraction to the internal event structure. Caregivers use language to help the child understand the sequence of the event, as in "we have to wash your hair first. Now let's rinse the soap out. Then we will get dry". These temporal words have no visual referent. Rather, they are learned by first perceiving a word that has no known meaning to the child. This process of acquiring meaning through context results in the acquisition of abstract language such as interpretations and inferences. [12] It also leads to greater complexity in discourse structures, as the child uses the words to discover temporal and causal links between actions within an event.

In this model, speech productions have an origin independent of the event structure, involving auditory and motor input and output. During infancy, the child's productions increasingly approximate the sounds of the language heard by the child. [18] During this phase, children with cleft palate would use compensatory strategies to best match the output to the input they heard. Children with better-developed event structures would make the transition from prelinguistic sounds productions such as babbling and jargon faster and more efficiently than children with fewer or more impoverished event structures. That is, the event structures have to be present to provide a context for mapping or learning language. These children would map the standard speech produced by others with event. The phonological rule system thus would develop consistent with this adult input. Once children had surgical repair of the palate, their speech productions would change to better match the accurate perceptions and phonological rules.

Children with fewer or more impoverished event structures would continue with prelinguistic sound productions longer. Further, without event structures they would have no context for mapping the speech produced by others with meaning. The compensatory productions would lack a meaningful context for change and therefore would become overlearned motor patterns. As event structures and the concomitant language were acquired, these learned productions would be incorporated into the phonological rule system. That is, the child would continue to match his established speech productions to the adult model. This would result in misperceptions of words and interfere with the processing of higher levels of language, or words learned within the event and linguistic context. CAD should thus contribute to maintaining the language delay. At the same time, the language delay and the incorporations of compensatory productions into the phonological rule system would serve to maintain CAD long after these speech modifications were physiologically necessary.

In fact, the children with CAD frequently demonstrate difficulty with both the event structures and the concomitant language. Many of the children could neither play productively with the toys nor interpret more than the most familiar early events (i.e., bathing) from pictures. Similarly, many times they do not demonstrate elaborated knowledge of events structures in the discourse analysis, marking neither temporal nor causal sequences of actions. Without the development of elaborated and complex event structures, a context for learning the language of interpretations and inferences would not be available. With these principles in mind, some methodologies for language and speech intervention suggest that language and speech should be presented in an integrated manner in order to introduce significant contexts for learning all linguistic elements.

Whole language is a teaching/learning philosophy that recognizes phonetic and phonology as an important component of a whole, assuming that language is indivisible. This teaching philosophy proposes that phonologic information should not be separated from the other areas of language, such as pragmatics or syntax. Thus, within the same activity, all areas of language, including phonology are provided. In this kind of intervention, the production of relevant speech sounds is taught and reinforced within communicative situations. Whole Language also validates some constructivist principles that guide the evaluation and intervention. [18] These principles suggest that children learn best when:

Language is used to talk about meaningful information and to accomplish purposes that make sense to the child; children are active participants in their own learning, not passive, quite listeners; learning involves repeated opportunities to interact and explore complex information; learning occurs in a context that is sensitive to the needs of individual children and that supports risk taking; language is "whole"; that is, it is presented in a context of meaning and use, not broken up and analyzed in small parts within an artificial setting; children use language to relate to one another and to become socialized as part of culture and community.

Treating only the CAD does not seem enough for these patients. It seems more appropriate to consider higher levels of language including abstract thought and reading and writing activities. In these contexts, phonologic information is integrated with all linguistic areas within communicative purposes and situations. In this order of ideas, the production of speech sounds is not the only goal. The goal is to become effective communicators. In this kind of intervention, the production of relevant speech sounds is taught and reinforced within communicative situations in relationship with higher organizational levels of language processing. [3] The use of abstract and complex levels of language that leads to a coherent and structured discourse can be facilitated in different teaching/learning contexts such as storybook reading. Storybooks are a perfect context for stimulating cognitive and language development in children. [12] Stories have all the elements of the narrative and discourse structure, including the relationships that provide order and structure such as temporality, causality or perspective. Also, they provide stability for seeing those relationships and for working on specific language needs such as articulation patterns of words and/or sounds. Other activities that promote working with speech and language in an integrated way are art, cooking, music or symbolic play.

Pamplona, et al, studied the rehabilitation of children with CAD within naturalistic contexts, following whole language teaching/learning philosophy principles. In this study, it was hypothesized that the most significant change would be concerning the phonologic system. This was not entirely true. Patients from the experimental group, who received therapy according to whole language philosophy, changed dramatically their overall language performance including their phonologic productions. All patients with CAD showed linguistic performance below the expected level according to chronological age. After the intervention period, besides phonologic improvement, children changed dramatically their overall language performance. [19]

STRATEGIES FOR ENHANCING PHONOLOGY

When intervention is based on the phonological principles, some implications for the assessment and management of children with cleft palate may be assumed, including analysis of phonologic processes in addition to phonetic analysis, and the use of facilitation strategies aimed to modify the phonologic system of each child.

The use of strategies seeks to scaffold the child's communicative turns to increase the child's speech and language performance. [3]

These strategies serve to assist the child in formulating messages with greater complexity, specificity of meaning, accuracy, and clarity of expression. Scaffolding strategies consists of various types of prompts, questions, information, restatements, and other procedures that provide support to the child as he/she is actively engaged in the process of communicating a message. [20]

Many phonologists have described specific strategies for facilitating a better way to communicate and/or articulate the sounds of speech. [2, 21] However, few of them have specified the expected time to apply each strategy in order to improve effectiveness. Some of the most common used strategies for are the following: Modeling, [3, 22] Phonemic Cues, [20] Minimal Pairs, [2, 23] Cycles, [21] Imitation and drills, [24] Requests for clarifications, [25] Phonetic changes, [20] and Expansions, [3] among others.

Phonological acquisition is gradual. [21, 26] It is a process. For assessment and intervention, it is important to understand the system of each child, and to recognize in which step of the process is at the moment. A clinical scale of severity of CAD in cleft palate children had been used for this purpose. [27] This scale describes what the child is doing and the difficulty he/she has to manage each specific sound of speech in order to correct placement and manner of articulation. This scale has been useful for understanding the specific moment in the process of each child. It also establishes the degree of severity of CAD in each patient, and facilitates setting intervention goals.

The scale mentioned herein is described as follows:

- •*Appropriate articulation.* The patient is able to produce adequate placement and manner of articulation during spontaneous speech, including non-present situations.

- *Inconsistent articulation.* The patient shows compensatory articulation errors inconsistently during spontaneous speech. Intelligibility is not significantly affected
- *Articulation within context.* The patient self-corrects articulation when using speech within a specific context. For example during telling a story from a story book which the patient already knows well. Nonetheless he shows frequent compensatory errors during spontaneous speech.
- *Articulation with strategies.* The patient can correct articulation during isolated words or selected short phrases, only when the clinician uses specific phonologic strategies.
- *Articulation of isolated phonemes.* The patient is able to correct articulation only in isolated phonemes through direct instruction.
- *Constant CAD.* The patient is not able to correct articulation not even in isolated phonemes and despite direct instruction.

Pamplona et al (2012), studied if some of the strategies commonly used in speech therapy for correcting compensatory articulation errors in children with cleft palate, could be more effective, depending on the degree of severity of CAD. In this study, the following strategies were used during speech therapy sessions: [28]

A. *Modeling:* Modeling is one of the most reported strategies. The speech pathologist models the speech and/or language behavior that the child is to learn. Some clinicians found that children respond spontaneously if the language behaviors being stressed are at the child's level. Thus, they model the behavior but do not normally request or formal elicitation. Modeling approaches the normal conditions of language learning more closely than the elicited imitation procedure. [22] Example: Child: "_all he_ (call her)". Clinician: "Yes, call her". This strategy has been often described as useful for language development, but it is also proposed as a phonologic strategy. Hoffman states that the models of appropriate articulated words in context are thought to help stimulate appropriate syllabic and phonemic organization. [3] The clinician has the opportunity to model and talk about the phonological structure of words within an overall communicative context. [29]
B. *Modeling with stress:* With this strategy, the speech pathologist models targeted sounds of speech, but includes a brief pause before

the sound and also, a stress on the sounds (phonemes) the clinician wants to model. [28] For example, during a play situation in which a cake is being cut, the child says "_ut the _ae_ (cut the cake); The clinician can respond "yes, (pause)....cut the (pause)...cake. I will (pause)...cut the (pause)...cake and give you a (pause)...piece".

C. *Cloze procedure with phonemic cues*: With this strategy, the clinician prompts the child's communicative turn by supplying part of the utterance and letting the child fill the rest. [30] If necessary, the clinician can provide the selected sound of the target word. [20] For example, when reading a storybook, the clinician can say: "Yes, she was hungry, and she found three bowls of sss ____ (soup) on the t t ____ (table)".
D. *Phonetic changes:* The speech pathologist indicates that the message would be more easily interpreted with a modification in speech production. [20] For example, when the child says "the _en (the pen)" reading a storybook in which there are different objects, the clinician says: "the pen". Remember to put your lips together and make an explosion: p p pen". With this strategy, the information would directly contribute to refining the phonemic distinction being articulated.
E. *Think aloud in phonemic awareness:* This is a metacognitive strategy where the speech pathologist verbalizes thoughts while reading a selection, thus modeling the process of comprehension. [31] This strategy enables to demonstrate the patient how to select an appropriate articulation process at a specific point in a particular communicative message. The clinician verbalizes specific think-aloud about different levels of Language organization including phonologic information. [28] For example, before reading a storybook, the clinician says: "Let us think which sounds we will be focusing on. We have to consider that some sounds are short and explosive like /k/, /p/, /t/. I will write these letters for reminding us to use them while we refer to the ideas and words of the book. Besides, we have other sounds that are long and continuous: /s/ or /f/. I will write these letters in this other paper. While looking at the storybook, the clinician is focusing on the target sounds and explaining the characteristics of each phoneme and how changing the sound can change the characteristics of the word increasing intelligibility.

For evaluation, all patients were recorded on videotape during speech therapy sessions and the methodology followed is called "narrative-centered themes". [18] This procedure provides naturally occurring contexts for acquiring world and everyday knowledge. It also serves as a means for addressing children's language and articulation, and allow for an extended exploration of a general concept. For this purpose, a main topic was chosen, and all activities were structured around this main topic. The goal was to work all linguistic areas in an integrated manner. Thus, articulation goals were always present in an organized whole. Most activities were realized as event representations such as play or storybook reading.

Children were divided in small groups depending on the age, linguistic development, and cognitive level.

All strategies were used within structured activities to provide children with contextually appropriate opportunities to use language and focus on articulation. The speech language pathologist (SLP) could choose either to expand an expression or refine upon an expressed idea by giving specific information, but anyway, SLP made sure that all strategies under study were used with each patient during the sessions.

SLP also used verbal expansions to provide children with information about higher levels of language organization. This type of interaction has been shown to increase the semantic and syntactic complexity of children's utterances, and could have similar effects upon children's phonological productions. [3]

All interactions were video recorded for later transcription and analysis. The examiners quantified the positive changes in articulation elicited by the use of each strategy. Positives changes were considered as the conditions in which the patients were able to approximate or correct appropriate placement or manner of articulation of the phonemes being used. The different strategies were compared in order to determine whether some strategies were more adequate for specific levels of severity of CAD.

Results demonstrated a significant relationship between effectiveness of all strategies and degree of severity of CAD in CCP. All the strategies yielded a significant higher number of positive modifications in articulation in patients classified in the milder levels of the scale, including patients with inconsistent compensatory errors during spontaneous speech and patients who were able to correct articulation within a familiar linguistic context. Moreover, there were a reduced number of positive changes in patients classified in the more severe levels, including patients who were able to correct compensatory errors during the production of words or short sentences, when they were being provided with specific instructions on placement and manner of articulation and patients who were able to correct compensatory errors only during the production of isolated phonemes, through direct instructions.

Hodson, who has largely contributed to the understanding of the phonologic principles in speech assessment and intervention, states that it is important to describe exactly what the child is doing, this allows providing a focus for more efficient remediation procedures. [21] Moreover, in order to achieve an efficient intervention, the SLP has to consider all the communicative emissions of the patient, including subtle changes in his/her speech during the interaction. This will allow the understanding of all linguistic rules interfering with the child's process for correcting articulation.

As a results of the study, strategies that included direct instruction such as phonetic change, cloze procedure with phonemic cues, and/or think aloud in phonemic awareness, appeared to be more effective for promoting positive changes in articulation in patients who were in the higher levels of severity of CAD, such as those who can only articulate correctly isolated phonemes or used them in words or short phrases with the support of the clinician. That is when these strategies were compared with those that do not include direct instruction such as modeling or modeling with stress, a significant difference was observed. However, these two strategies showed similar effectiveness in the lower levels of severity of articulation. In such levels, children articulate better and are more aware of the use of speech sounds, and show confidence for producing these sounds during a more structured discourse.

It is important to emphasize that modeling is one of the most frequent strategies described. [2, 3, 20] Also, the two strategies that included modeling -modeling and modeling with stress-, were the most common strategies used by the speech pathologists in the study. The results showed that these strategies do not seem to be as effective as the ones that include direct instruction when they are used in children with higher levels of severity of CAD. This finding has important implications for speech intervention. The clinician should consider the characteristics and level of severity of articulation impairment before deciding which strategy should be used.

It should be pointed out, that in the study, for speech intervention, different activities were structured in order to facilitate changes in the phonologic system of each child. Some of them had a structured context such as storybook reading/telling where the text or illustrations provided concrete information with visual cues to refer to. Also, talking about a graphic organizer was considered a structured and present context. In contrast, communicating during symbolic play situations in which the context or situation for playing had to be created with words, or talking about a non-present situation, were considered less structured linguistic context or event, since there were no visual cues supporting communication. In these instances, the individual has to create the whole context through language (decontextualized situation). When the positive changes in articulation elicited by the use of the strategies mentioned above, were compared in more structured and less structured contexts, there seemed to be similar positive changes in both situations. Nonetheless, when the strategies that do not include direct instruction on articulation such as modeling, or modeling with stress were being assessed, there seemed to be a tendency for more positive changes when the strategies were being used in more structured contexts, such as storybook reading / telling. This finding can be explained since these structured situations can provide more contextual or concrete support for communication. This can be especially relevant for the higher levels of severity of CAD, and speech pathologists should consider it for intervention. Moreover, when children with articulation errors are treated, providing visual support is a valuable tool for scaffolding.

In a later study, Pamplona and colleagues studied the efficacy of the strategies for treating CA in CCP. [32] In this occasion they compared two different ways for using scaffolding strategies during intervention in CCP. Both groups received speech therapy aimed to correct compensatory articulation according to the principles of the Whole Language Model where storybook readings were the main context for intervention. Intervention was aimed to reinforce correct speech sounds while enhancing cognitive linguistic organization.

Within these main principles of intervention, in the first group (control group), the SLP used the strategies described before for phonologic intervention. The SLP was instructed that all strategies should be attempted in each case. In contrast, in the second group (experimental group) the SLP used the same phonologic strategies, but they were selected according with the level of severity of CAD as assessed by the scale described herein. [28] (See table 1). When comparing the levels of advance in both groups, a Mann Whitney test showed a significant difference that indicates a greater advance in the experimental group. In conclusion, considering the characteristics of the phonologic system of each child can be useful for facilitating the selection of some strategies, which may be more effective than others in any particular case. Moreover, the dynamics involved in each strategy were analyzed. Some strategies appeared to be more appropriate for different stages in the natural process of correcting a compensatory articulatory pattern in CCP.

Table 1. Use of strategies according to the level of severity of CAD

Level of articulation	Characteristics of the level The patient:	Strategies
Constant CA	Is not able to correct articulation not even in isolated phonemes and despite direct instruction.	Phonetic changes, Think aloud in PA.
Articulation in isolated phonemes	Is able to correct articulation only in isolated phonemes through direct instruction.	Phonetic changes, Cloze proc with PC, Think aloud in PA
Articulation with strategies	Can correct articulation during isolated words or selected short phrases, only with support of the clinician.	Phonetic changes, Cloze proc with PC, Think aloud in PA, Modeling with stress.
Articulation within context	Self-corrects articulation within a specific context. Shows frequent CA errors during spontaneous speech.	Modeling with stress, Modeling.
Inconsistent articulation	Shows CA errors inconsistently during spontaneous speech.	Modeling with stress, Modeling.
Appropriate articulation	Is able to produce adequate placement and manner of articulation during spontaneous speech.	

The results of these two studies suggest that when speech strategies are used according to the severity of the compensatory articulatory pattern (which is classified depending on the frequency of its appearance during speech and the response to correction prompts), it seems easier for the child to follow the speech pathologist lead in order to correct the pattern.

Patients who are able to produce a correct articulatory pattern only on isolated phonemes or short words, with consistent prompting are more likely to show an effective response to direct instruction on placement and manner of articulation. A possible explanation is that these patients show a limited level of phonologic awareness. In contrast, strategies, which use modeling and modeling with stress seem to be effective in patients with lower degrees of severity of CAD. These patients appear to be more aware of the characteristics of the speech sounds.

It can be concluded that selecting the speech pathology treatment strategies for each case, according with its specific characteristics, including the severity of the articulation disorder, as assessed by its use in conversational speech and the response to prompting, can become a valuable procedure for improving outcome during speech intervention.

INTERVENTION

Considering that language is indivisible, and that learning occurs from whole to part to whole, intervention should treat all areas of language within meaningful contexts according to the child's level of development. These contexts are based in more / less familiar events and allow focusing on the target sounds and language structure or organization.

The intention is to create a natural environment for language learning. The activities have to be carefully designed to be consistent with whole language principles of learning where language is an integral part of every activity. The lessons are organized to help children make sense of complex information while they acquire and use language. This allows CCP to focus on speech and language learning while they do interesting and fun activities.

One strategy is to expose children to a wide variety of books some which include a repeatable and predictable text, others that have great and explicit drawings, and finally, others which challenge listening and critical thinking abilities because of their more complex and abstract story and/or content. It is described that storybooks are great for stimulating cognitive and language development in children. [18] Storybooks have all the elements of the narrative and discourse structure, including the relationships that provide order and structure such as temporality, causality or perspective. Also, the information in the illustrations and the language used in context provide stability for seeing those relationships and for working on specific language needs such as articulation patterns of words and/or sounds. For children with CAD, having both, visual and phonologic information in a simultaneous way can enhance better results. [28]

Other activities that promote working with speech and language are art, play, cooking, and music.

STORYBOOK READING

Strategies

In order to choose the right storybook each child has to be carefully evaluated to get to know his/her linguistic level and phonologic preferences. Knowing the system of each child allows the SLP to interact in an adequate level according to his/her developmental characteristics.

During storybook reading the different aspects of language that required special attention in CCP must be addressed. At the beginning, the story and the illustrations give context for constructing meaning by talking about the actions, characters or sequence of the story. Repeated readings or redundant ideas are useful for understanding and organizing the information as it become familiar. These familiar contexts will facilitate focusing in articulation in a meaningful way while acquiring complex and structured language. In other words, the story is the whole that will allow working with patterns or specific sounds, and then these specific parts will be integrated again in the whole. By modifying the child's internalized rules governing production, the child's speech changes to match this revised category. Because the phonological rule is integrated with other aspects of language, occurrence of correct sounds in spontaneous production is more rapid. [20] The sound does not first have to be learned as a motor production and then generalized to language and spontaneous speech. All areas of language work together as a complex system moving into integration.

Different strategies must be used during storybook reading. These strategies can be used before, during and after reading in order to provide tools for constructing meaning and focusing in specific parts such as the sounds of speech.

Before reading, activating prior knowledge or predicting about the story can help to focus on meaning and start constructing the topic. Also, talking about the target sounds is useful for developing awareness and get ready for articulating during the task.

During the storybook reading two major goals are to be established. First, pay attention to the structure and content of the story for enhancing linguistic organization, and second, to practice and work with the target sounds in articulation. For linguistic organization helping the children to follow the story and make connections, predictions, interpretations or inferences in order to help them see the relationships and conclusions. For articulation, using strategies like the mentioned before or focusing on the target sounds by analyzing words or patterns could help the child to match events with words and sounds for improving articulation and developing phonemic awareness. This would facilitate generalization into connected speech. Finally, after the storybook reading, many activities for responding to the story can be developed such as: use/make graphic organizers for analyzing the narrative structure of the story (beginning, problem, end); analyzing a character or the setting; analyzing feelings, solutions; making art or representing the story or parts of the story. This will allow focusing on articulation as the topic becomes familiar by reading, analyzing and talking about it. During the whole reading, emphasizing the target sounds would allow to hear those sounds in a context of use and develop awareness about their contribution for creating meaning.

Many authors who follow phonologic principles recommend a set of strategies aimed to facilitate changes in phonologic processes. Some of these strategies are based on phonologic development in infants and toddlers. Some of these strategies are to be used during intervention for enhancing stimulation in CCP and CAD. Hodson, in 1991 stated that children with highly unintelligible speech can discriminate others productions, but seem to discount their own auditory feedback signals, even when hearing is judged to be within normal limits. The author suggests providing auditory stimulation during speech therapy sessions for enhancing the development of this ability. [21] This auditory stimulation can be provided if the sounds are stressed and identified during the storybook reading. The purpose is to help the child to rely on auditory feedback and metalinguistic knowledge while following the structure and information of the story and illustrations. In this process, self-monitoring skills are enhanced.

Ingram, studied phonologic development. He described that children learn best the sounds that are necessary to their language, and these sounds are the ones that appears frequently. [26] Modifying linguistic context in order to make the target sounds appear frequently can help children to focus on those sounds and practice articulation while following the plot or event.

Conclusion

In conclusion, working articulation within a linguistic whole may be a perfect context for intervention with CCP. Naturalistic contexts such as play or story telling allow for event structures and related language to be examined for semantic context, discourse organization and situational representation while focusing on the sounds of speech.

In these situations, selecting the speech pathology treatment strategies for each case, according with its specific characteristics, including the severity of the articulation disorder, as assessed by its use in conversational speech and the response to prompting, can become a valuable procedure for improving outcome during the speech intervention.

References

[1] Norris, J. & Damico, J. (1990). Whole language in theory and practice: implication for language intervention. *Language Speech and Hearing Services in Schools*, 21, 212-220.

[2] Fey, M. (1992) Clinical Forum: Phonological Assessment and Treatment. Articulation and Phonology: An Introduction. *Language, Speech and Hearing Services in Schools*, 23, 224-232. Vol 32, Number 2.

[3] Hoffman. P. (1992). Clinical Forum: Phonological Assessment and Treatment. Synergistic Development of Phonetic Skill. *Language, Speech and Hearing Services in Schools* 23, 254-260.

[4] McWilliams, B., Morris, H. & Shelton, R. (1990). Cleft palate speech (2nd ed.) Philadelphia: BC Decker.

[5] Pamplona, M. Ysunza, A., Guerrero, M., Mayer, I. & Garcia-Velasco, M. (1996). Surgical correction of velopharyngeal insufficiency with and without compensatory articulation. *Int. J. of Pediatric Otorhinolaryngol,* 34, 53-59.

[6] Pamplona, M., Ysunza, A. & Espinoza, J. (1999). A Comparative trial of two modalities of speech intervention for compensatory articulation in cleft palate children, phonologic approach versus articulatory approach. *Int. J of pediatric otorhinolaryngology*, 49, 21-26.

[7] Kuehn, DP & Moller, KT. (2000). Speech and language issues in the cleft palate population: the state of the art. *Cleft Palate Craniofac J.* 37, 1-35.

[8] Bzoch, K. R. (1965) Articulation proficiency and error patterns of preschool cleft palate and normal children. *Cleft Palate J.* 2, 340-349.

[9] McDonald, E.T. (1964) Articulation Testing and Treatment: A sensory-motor approach, Pittsburgh PA: Stanwix-House.

[10] Chapman, K. (1993) Phonologic processes in children with cleft palate. *Cleft Palate J.* 30, 64-71.

[11] Hoffman, P. & Daniloff, R. (1990). Evolving Views of Children's Disordered Speech Sound Production from Motoric to Phonological. *JSLPA/ROA,* 14, 13-22

[12] Norris, J. & Hoffman, P. (1993). Whole language intervention for school-age children. San Diego, CA: Singular Publishing Group.

[13] Hardin-Jones, M & Champan, K. (2011). Cognitive and Language Issues Associated with Cleft Lip and Palate. *Seminars in Speech Lang*, 32, 127–140.

[14] Powers, G. (1990). Speech analysis of four children with repaired cleft palate. *Journal of Speech and Hearing Disorders*, 55, 542-550.

[15] Young, Pourcel, & Ballard. (2010). Expressive language skills in Chinese Singaporean preescholers with nonsyndromic cleft lip and/or palate. *International Journal of Pediatric Otorhinolaryngology*, 74:456-464.

[16] Pamplona, M., Ysunza, A., González, M., Ramírez, E., & Patiño, C. (2000). Linguistic development in cleft palate patients with and without compensatory articulation disorder. *International journal of Otorhinolaryngology*, 54, 81-91.

[17] Damico, J. (1992). Systematic observation of communicative interaction: A valid and practical descriptive assessment technique. In W.A. Secord & J.S. Damico (Eds.), Best practices in school speech-language pathology. San Antonio, TX: Psychological Corp, Pp 133-144.

[18] Norris, J. & Hoffman, P. (1995). Storybook-Centered Themes. Tucson, Arizona: Communication Skill Builders.

[19] Pamplona, M, Ysunza, A, & Ramírez, P. (2004). Naturalistic intervention in cleft palate children. *International Journal of Pediatric Otorhynolaryngology*, 68, 75-81.

[20] Norris, J. & Hoffman, P. (1990). Language intervention within naturalistic environments. *Language, Speech and Hearing Services in Schools*, 21, 72-84.

[21] Hodson, B and Paden, E. (1993). Targeting Intelligible Speech. San Diego, CA: College Hill Press.

[22] Bloom, L. & Lahey, M. (1978). Language development & language disorders. New York: John Wiley & Sons.

[23] Gierut, J. (1989). Maximal opposition approach to phonological treatment. *Journal of Speech and Hearing Disorders*, 54, 9-19.

[24] Elbert, M & Gierut, J. (1986). Handbook of clinical phonology: Approaches to assessment and treatment, New York: College-Hill Press.

[25] Wollner, S., Geller, E. (1984). Methods for assessing pragmatic abilities. In J.V. Irwin (Ed.), Pragmatics: The role in language development (pp. 135-160). La Verne, CA: Fox Point.

[26] D. Ingram. (1976). Phonological disability in children. New York: Elsevier.

[27] Pamplona, M., Ysunza, A., Patiño, C., Ramírez, E., Drucker, M., Mazón, J. (2005). Speech summer camp for treating articulation disorders in cleft palate patients. *Int. J. of Pediatric Otorhynolaryngology*, 69, 351-359.

[28] Pamplona, M., Ysunza, A., Chavelas, K., Aramburu, E., Patiño, C., Martí, F. (2012) Strategies for providing Speech Therapy in patients with cleft palate and compensatory articulation errors. *Journal of Maxillofacial and Oral Surgery*. Vol 11, Number 2, 11,144-151.

[29] Hoffman, P. (1990). Spelling, phonology, and the speech language pathologist: A whole language perspective. *Language, Speech, and Hearing Services in Schools*, 21, 238-243.

[30] Snow, CD., Nathan, D. & Pearlman, R. (1985). Assessing children's knowledge about book reading. In L. Galda & A. Pellegrini (Eds.). Play and stories, Nerwood, NJ: Ablex.

[31] Palinscar, AS & Brown, AL. (1985). Reciprocal teaching of comprehension-fostering and monitoring activities. *Cognition and Instruction*, I, 117-175.

[32] Pamplona, M., Ysunza, A. & Morales, S. (2014). Strategies for treating compensatory articulation in children with cleft palate. *International journal of Biomedical Science*. 10(1), 43-51.

INDEX

C

D

E

F

L

M

N

O

P

Q

R

S

T

U

V

W

Y